Tension Management :

Techniques, Approaches & Strategies

Navin K. Kalra
Alka Kalra

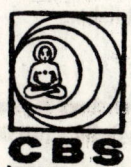

CBS

CBS PUBLISHERS & DISTRIBUTORS

4596/1A, 11 DARYAGANJ NEW DELHI - 110 002

ISBN : 81-239-0438-X

First Edition : 1996
Reprint : 2004

Published by:

Satish Kumar Jain for CBS Publishers & Distributors
4596/1A, 11 Darya Ganj, New Delhi - 110 002 (INDIA)

Printed at :
Asia Printograph, Shahdara, Delhi - 110 032 (India)

FOREWORD

The present volume is an outcome of intensive reading and extensive experience of bearing tension and strain by Mr. Navin K Kalra and Dr. Alka Kalra since 1987.

An accident resulted in a queer disability to the left leg of the male author but propelled and prompted the couple – Dr. Alka Kalra and Mr. Navin K. Kalra, to think of studying the phenomena of tension, stress and anxiety and of preparing a book on coping with tension and understanding the various techniques, approaches and modalities of controlling and overcoming the tension, both physical and psychological.

The term tension has been widely used to describe a number of situations in which an individual, a group or a community finds itself at times. This word has also been used to denote the emotional motivations and cognitive states of the individual or the group which may persist over a period of time and give rise to a variety of unusual patterns of behaviour. Examining the manifold contexts and the writings in which this ubiquitous term has been used, one finds that like any other attractive and extensively used word, tension is not a well defined term.

In the writings of the psychologists, tension is used to refer to two different but interdependent states. Sometimes this word is used to describe the emotional and cognitive state of a single organism and sometimes it refers to the emotional, motivational and cognitive state shared by a group of individuals in their interactions with another group. The first connotation of tension has been of much use in explaining learning, vigilance, goal-directed activity, frustration, conflict, psychoneurotic and psycho-somatic disorders. The second is used in the context of intergroup relations and implies prejudices, stereotypes, intolerance, distrust and even outbursts of violence.

In the present volume, the authors have covered a wide canvas. After considering the nature and genesis of tension, an attempt has been made to identify the roots of tension and to explain a variety of factors of individual tension. All important types of strategies and therapies for coping with individual tension have been described and discussed, specially philosophical, psychological, physical (relaxation) and medical approaches and techniques have been enumerated and analysed. The book provides a comprehensive frame for analysis and understanding of individual tension and explains its possible and probable causes. The authors deserve my hearty congratulations for writing this book in a lucid and systematic style, without using cumbersome jargon. Hopefully, this book will serve a useful purpose in the understanding and controlling of individual tension.

Joe Khatena
Professor & Head
Department of Educational Psychology
Mississipi State University
Mississipi (United States)

PREFACE

In the competitive world of today there is need to utilise one's energy to get optimum results. One should not dissipate his/her energy to get unrealistic results. Because of din and clamour of modern life, one finds a latent sense of dismay and frustration in people. The materialistic pursuit of deriving hedonistic and sensuous pleasure has left an emptiness which has engulfed people from all angles, rendering them incapable of healthy living, positive thinking and spiritual awakening.

Tension is an ailment directly related to fast pace of life in the scientific and technological age of today. These days even at home a person's 'life/fate' is sealed between the telephone and the alarm clock. As tension is part of a man's life, everyone has to learn more and more about coping with and controlling of tension. Though as a part of the competitive environment around, none can get rid of tension and its evil influences but there is always a possibility to use one's knowledge of making that harmful energy work positively for him. To maintain oneself in the state of desired degree of objectivity it is necessary to understand the various facets of the term "tension". Modern life presents various physical, mental and emotional challenges for which it is necessary for a person to be relaxed and tension-free.

This book is an attempt to explain the ways to attain well being through the open door of tension. Tension is so intimately interwoven with every social creature's life that while its effects are far-reaching, many a time it remains unnoticeable. This volume is intended to be a guidance source for the common man to have insight into the problems of tension. It tries to help a person to live a better life, full of happiness and make it more productive. This book presents and explains tension management techniques which are really effective in a life full of hassles and heavy pressures. As people vary in their tolerance of tension, the effects of tension also vary from minor diseases to premature deaths. Through this book multiphasic tension is introduced to show its effects on human body and mind and to give an interesting programme of controlling the severe effects, only by making one conscious of the value of the unnoticeable factors in many walks of life. It depicts the bird's eye view of tension spectrum and provides a guidance programme for enjoying a healthy life. It also lays stress on a multi approach solution for handling the problems of tension through a variety of approaches : Medical approach, Psychological approach, Food habits, Spiritual approach, Physical activity approach and such other modalities. The authors have developed an insight to understand the effects of alcoholism, smoking and sexual relations on tension and have suggested the ways and means of getting maximum benefit by using the various relaxation techniques such as yoga, meditation, hypnotism and the like. In modern times, tensions in day-to-day life are increasing. Man is madly running towards achieving materialistic goals. The traditional thinking of using intellect towards worldy things and faith in spiritual matters has almost got a reversal. This reversal in thinking has led people to use the intellect in spiritual matters and faith in worldly things.

The so called father of stress research, Selye, (1980) has rightly said : "Stress suffers from the mixed blessing of being too well known or too little understood". It is basically an individual's experience of fluctuating range of psychic or mental state. It is nothing but a stimulus or a condition that produces demand in human beings to exceed their ordinary level of functioning or to work below the usual level of functioning.

To adapt oneself effectively to a tension producing environment, it is necessary to be conscious of what this term stands for and what its effects are on one's body and mind. The emotional and psychological burden created by the system of human body is termed as tension. Energy when harnessed properly can create wonders but when this gets misdirected it can create devastating effects. The effects are not only physical or mental but can be emotional also. The evil effects get reflected in the form of various symptoms when the body fails to give cushion to absorb its shocking effects. This body, a wonderful complexity provided by Almighty, provides enough danger signals for a man to understand and analyse. Alas! such signals don't get their due importance in our hectic life-style.

This book not only provides insight for understanding the problems of tension but also helps in understanding the body language, its danger signals and symptoms that are reflected. The problem of tension can corrode anyone irrespective of his caste, colour or religion. This book beautifully provides practical strategies and coping mechanisms that can be adopted to overcome it in a good way. It provides a multi-dimensional approach to this multi-phasic problem. The topics covered touch one's day to day life activities which are normally missed out by our conscious mind.

This book makes an attempt to describe and discuss the various techniques and approaches that can help to tackle the menace of tension. Special emphasis has been laid on tension from three angles viz. philosophical, psychological and physiological. Under philosophical approach, the authors have given the gist of the teachings of religious scriptures of various philosophies which are well known all over the world for giving direction to peace-seekers. The authors have worked hard to cover various relevant topics under the psychological and physiological approaches. Besides, the authors have covered different systems of medical care that can be relied upon to tackle the problem of tension. The various curative and preventive approaches discussed in this book open a gateway for the readers to explore further to handle tension in the best possible way within their environmental constraints. The most interesting part of the book includes practical tips provided by the authors which they applied during the tense periods of their life.

Navin K. Kalra
Alka Kalra

CONTENTS

1

INTRODUCTION

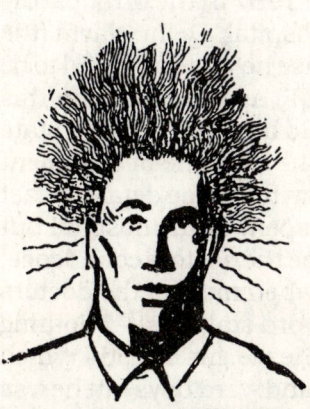

BACKGROUND AND RATIONALE

Modern society is stressful. The life of every individual is full of events, oddities and eventualities that create stress, anxiety and depression. Through healthy management techniques and sound coping strategies one can maintain mental poise and overcome distress. There is no need to become an escapist or a deranged man. One should face the hard and harsh realities of personal and social life bravely, and boldly and resolve the problems imaginatively and meticulously. There is a need to restore normalcy and acquire "psychological balance" through knowledge and understanding, experience and imagination, and will and wisdom.

All of us, being a part of this human society face and experience tension. Furthermore, each individual has learnt and adopts different strategies for coping with the problems created by stress.

Some try to follow escapism while others adopt avoidism. Actually we all have an organ called "brain" in our body which helps us to tackle these problems. Some of us use it to a great deal, others don't use it much. It is not that who use their brain always have ready solutions for all the problems but it also depends upon how much information one has regarding the problem and its solutions. Yes, dear reader, this book is to make you aware of alternatives as and when you need them. The authors led a normal life before the tragic road accident. The accident resulted in tension and gradually they overcame it through insight and experience, study and imagination, and medication and therapy. There is no person who is free from tension, stress, anxiety and the resultant depression.

*   *   *   *   *   *

It was the morning of April 21, 1987 in the orthopaedic ward of Dr. Ram Manohar Lohia Hospital, Delhi. Navin (the male author), was little upset because he was supposed to be referred to a different hospital (LNJP) as the doctors in this hospital felt that nothing much could be done with that state of health. He was doubtful about the new line of treatment as the new doctors must not be knowing all the details of last four months of injured life that he spent in the hospital but he was hopeful, on the contrary to see the doctors confidence, to accept him at such a bad state when most of the doctors refused the case by saying a three word statement– "Nothing can be done!". He was stirred to leave his friends which included patients, doctors, nurses and ward boys but he was stimulated to accept the change because at times it was very boring to see the same walls and curtains and the same beds and those white bedsheets. It was more than four months since he saw a flower smiling on a plant, grass on the land, children playing and yelling. He had gone little emotional when since morning one by one each of his friends who were working in the hospital, right from a stretcher carrying person to the x-ray specialist came to say "bye" and "good health". He found other patients looking at his side with a mixed feeling. They were happy to see him going away for better treatment, on the other hand they were sad to lose a friend who could joke around with them and discuss lively issues.

He was on his bed and watching Alka, (the female author) doing the final packing of the things which were with them for the last four months. Finally a word came "Ambulance is ready". He took a deep breath and smiled. He was taken from his bed to the ambulance, Wow! What an experience!. He felt the air had lovely fragrance outside, he could breath smoothly. When he looked at road side, he felt for last four months his world was very small, every thing looked so different–a bus, a road, the people, the traffic lights and even the small birds could attract him towards them. He found the world full of lovely creatures, every thing was soothing to his eyes. But suddenly his attention was drawn when he saw people running in cars, buses and so on. He felt in his life there is a small gap, he was still for a time being but is running very fast and in this competitive run he had lost full four months. Though this thought could have brought depression but he reasoned out :

Is everybody running constructively ? Most of the people who are running today are not thinking of themselves; some of them are running against desired direction. At least he was not running. He was motionless for time being but he can use this time constructively, to plan his run as soon a⅃ he will be out on the roads. Yes, dear readers this book is that planning which we could do not only for ourselves but for our dear friends like you who are so busy that though they are capable but they don't get time to plan something for their own GOOD HEALTH.

* * * * *

The main motivation of writing this book is to make the readers think and become aware of the concept of 'Tension' which is fast invading their life. Unless the so-called symptoms are properly handled in time, the same can create havoc. The authors had vivid glimpses of the effects of tension. Navin Kalra, the first author, met with a road accident on 12th January, 1987 and had to be in the hospital for six months with full length plaster on his left leg for about two years. He met with a minor accident but ignorance and innocence of doctors and patient resulted in such a delayed recovery. Even today ill-effects are continuing. The authors would like to share the experiences of the accident period which they had undergone at a young age of 29 years and that too within nine months of their marriage.

Navin, (the male author) can recollect with pride the active life he had led. He had the privilege to be the captain of his school cricket team. He used to have daily walk/run for 10 kilometers. He had formal two months training in Karate and had been a very active instructor of Bhartiya Yoga Sansthan, New Delhi since 1981. He is a Chartered Accountant by profession whose life before the accident used to start at 4.15 a.m. and he could be seen in formal dress with neck tie right from 7.00 a.m. to 10.00 p.m. His busy hectic schedule included various activities including involvement that was demanded by his profession and also on account of being actively associated with Lions Club, Delhi Fort. He had seen contrast of yoga life vis-a-vis late night party life.

It is a known fact that human beings are the most developed species on this earth in the sense that all the credit for miracles go to them. The miracle of technology and wonders of architecture, the beauty of art, dance and music, all are the products of man's genius. But dear reader, have you ever given enough thought to understand the importance of each of your body organ which are the creations of His wonders. Here experience speaks, when Navin was confined to bed for long time due to the leg injury, the doctors were equally worried about the other parts of the body to keep them fit through exercises, which normally one does not realise. All the human body parts like lungs, kidneys, heart and others automatically work with normal day-to-day activity. Navin was asked by the doctors to blow up a football bladder every day to maintain the capacity of lungs to retain sufficient oxygen and to do bullworker exercise to keep shoulders and muscles of hand in order. Confinement to bed slows down the working of various parts of the body. The anger and aggression is directly related to ones physical strength was realized by Navin in the hospital.

Life is not in one's own hand. Destiny has its own role to play but leaving everything on destiny is not a correct approach. Belief in Karma-Yoga is worth pursuing. Navin, at very young age decided to have drug-free natural life and as such he was regularly taking exercises to keep him fit, but two years of confinement to bed made him to have heavy dosage of medicines beyond his wishes, intention and imagination.

It was usual to share pleasantly jokes with minimum of fifty to eighty persons daily. It has been realised that if one has known five real caring friends, it is something marvellous. The value of real friendship was experienced first time in life after the accident. There is no grudge or grouse with the rest of the seventy friends who are busy in this materialistic world but feel bad for taking long time in realising the greatness of those five caring friends.

*   *   *   *   *

One fine Friday morning 11'o clock, Navin decided to leave the orthopaedic ward of LNJP Hospital, New Delhi. He decided this so suddenly, that too immediately after the doctor's routine round to the ward. Alka, the second author the wife of the patient, was surprised to hear such decision of Navin, the justification of such quick decision keeping in view the bad state of left leg was beyond her imagination and rational thinking. She curiously and tactfully tried to know the reason of such a hasty decision. Navin told that today he has been declared drug addict by the senior doctor of the team "Drug Addict!", that was Alka's immediate response. She could not understand how a person who does not smoke, drink or habitually enjoy any intoxicants could be declared "Drug Addict" by a team of highly qualified doctors. To be true, he had developed drug dependence. The doctors had learnt that he was daily taking four to five pain killers to overcome his breath-taking pain in the right leg (other than the fractured left leg).

Navin had continuous rolling tears after the visit of the doctors. Keeping in view that Navin had never such irrational reaction in the last five months of hospitalisation, Alka was suprised and wanted to know the details of the discussion he had with the doctors. He was told that his pain was only psychological and it did not have any identified physical symptoms. Navin's tension was built-up because he was having intolerable pain in his right leg.

Later Alka explored the problem from doctors who reviewed the condition of the left and right legs and concluded that Navin was suffering from bone infection in the thigh of the right leg which was very painful but pain-killer had bad side-effect, which was bad for him otherwise. The infection in the left leg was more than the right and with the help of medicines doctors were trying to treat the infection. Another operation in such stage was not advisable. As they were helpless and they certainly wanted Navin to stop taking too many pain killers every day. They thought of colouring the problem to be psychological.

Out of this incident it can be concluded that when the things do not move in the desired direction, tension is created and it builds up. The discrepancy in the thinking process of one individual or difference of opinion between two can cause serious tension. As Navin was tense due to difference of opinion among the senior doctors who were acting out to prove that there was no pain.

*   *   *   *   *

The first author, Navin can mention with pride that he faced tension with patience for 8 years and to a good extent recovered without amputation. The reason of his fast and excellent recovery was that he had never allowed the tension to over-rule him. Through this book we share our tried and tested methods of tension removal, wich helped us all through. We want to tell the readers all the aspects of tension so that when need arises people are in a position to choose the best option for them. Before one understand the management aspects let us visualise the total picture of tension starting from causes and its bad effects on the human body.

The causes of the tension can broadly be explained under the following three headings :

(i) **Environmental causes** : These are solely external factors existing in the individual's physical world e.g. drugs, noise, humidity, temperature variations, chemical pollutants, flood and the like.

(ii) **Social causes** : These are externally induced and result from interaction of the individual with his environment. e.g. death of a loved one, retirement, divorce, these are negative stressors which create distress, and marriage ceremonies, engagement etc. are positive stressors which normally create eustress.

(iii) **Self induceed :** These are the most damaging ones due to their recurrent nature. To a great extent their intensification depends on the individual's personality make-up, e.g. frustration, guilt, worry, anger, resentment, inferiority, self-pity, etc.

Different individuals react differently to different situations. Behaviour and mood of a person is not only dependent on present situation; but is deeply affected by one's hope, desire, wish, and how one sees his own accumulated experience of the past. Competence to deal with tension differs from individual to individual depending on their emotional reactions, persistence, flexibility and degree of ego-defensiveness.

Effects of Tension

The effects of tension can be either short term or long term.

A. **Short-term effects :** These are less intense and last for shorter periods of time. Effects can be broadly studied under four heads as follows :

(a) Behavioural effects : These effects can be observed in an individual due to changing behaviour, e.g. over-eating or excessive consumption of tea, coffee, etc.

(b) Emotional effects : The individual undergoing tension shows heightened anxiety, depression or anger.

(c) Cognitive Effects : The person affected by tension shows increased distractibility and decreased concentration on any task.

(d) Physiological effects : The organism feels rapid heart beat, high/low blood pressure and heightened muscle tension.

B. **Long term effects :** These effects are more damaging and stay for longer period. These are very intense and disease producing. These long term effects can again be studied under the following four heads :

(a) Behavioural disorders : The individual under heightened tension shows the symptoms of obesity and alcoholism.

(b) Emotional disorders : The individual shows chronic anxiety. depression, phobia, mental illness etc.

(c) Cognitive disorders : The individual shows the symptoms of memory loss, sleep disorders and problems of obsessive thoughts.

(d) Physiological disorders : The individual undergoes severe headaches, hypertension and heart diseases.

Some of the general ways of dealing with tension include –

(i) To remove unwanted causes of tension from one's life.

(ii) Not to allow certain events to become 'tension provoking'.

(iii) To develop technique to handle tension so that it leads to least possible bad effects.

(iv) To increase capacity to bear the tension demand by seeking relaxation and by diversion to pleasure giving habits.

Tension can be handled among other approaches by relaxation techniques.

The technique of Shavasana, auto-suggestion and meditation was tried in hospital but perhaps failed in reaching the indepth stage of the same. From this, an important principle can be derived that one's intake of food and medicine affects the functioning of mind. For meditation, it is important to take care of the food.

One can succeed in handling the tension created particularly during the period of hospitalisation by adopting the following techniques :

1. **By diversion of mind** : To keep oneself busy in reading books and listening to music/songs. It was realised that diversion of mind can be more effective if pursuit is made with curiosity on account of information gap, i.e. knowledge one intends to have and information one actually has. This leads one to involve himself more deeply.

2. **By Pranayama** : During confinement to bed it was

found that Pranayana played effective role in keeping the spirit high.

3. **Limited physical activity :** Though at the time of exercise various organs of the body are under tension but the after effects of exercise are too good if the same is undertaken within permissible limit. This helps in elimination organs to work effectively, digestive system and other systems get activated leading to creation of more energy.

4. **Acting :** The habit of saying "I am fine" initially more or less in a mechanical way also helps. This masking of bad emotions and always saying "I am fine" was taken by the first author from father in particular. This typical acting for creation of good expression on the face even in odd situations, does help in reducing the bad effects of tension. It can be realised that it is necessary to rise above the situation rather than getting bogged down into the problem. The initial artificiality in this regard may result in creating pleasant effect.

It is recollected that once in the hospital when there was energy even to create an audible word how was tension overcome and confidence regained. His eyes were closing down. There was a feeling of breathlessness. This was realised by the friends and relatives. They rushed to a doctor and called him from hostel as it was Sunday and doctors on duty were available only in emergency. A doctor was requested and persuaded to examine the patient. The friends who were available at that time thought perhaps only the last limited breaths to live had arrived. The doctor came and he asked "Mr. Kalra, how are you?" To this, the usual response was "Fine". This answer was never expected by the friends and the doctor but such an automatic reply which was more or less mechanical helped in recovering fast and in maintaining high spirit in a strange tressful situation.

5. **Keep yourself engaged :** Another way of keeping oneself busy is to read lot many books particularly in the field of stress and tension. An idea of writing

a book was instantaneously born and today the idea has turned out in reality. It has been realised that when one keeps oneself busy in useful aversions the physical pain can be forgotten. The idea of writing a book on tension by the patient was really appreciated by a practising orthopaedician of a foreign country who came to the hospital at the instance of one of his friends. He very wittingly summarised his advice "Mr. Kalra, keep yourself engaged and involved in something, it does not matter even if you are busy on tension" (subject of the book).

6. **Being optimistic :** It can be tried to be optimistic possibly all the time. Even the firm and final advice of amputation of the leg in black and white by a leading orthopaedician did not disturb or led to fear. It is always good to think positively. It is felt that the left leg has recovered to a great extent but sttill it is far from normal. The associated nerves have been badly affected in this process by which the author is unable to have control over the movement of his left leg, fingers and toes. There is shortage of time to take care of his left leg due to his social and family commitment, otherwise it is felt that strong will-power and use of the therapy of auto-suggestion, the powers of nerves can be possibly be restored. Even the recovery can be made faster but one is bound by the circumstances of so many things which are easy to say but much difficult to practise and money has its own role to play.

7. **Feeling of success :** By concentration on areas where one achieves success, the feeling of happiness can be created. It is necessary to have taste of success if you are unsuccessful as continuous failures can make one depressed.

To test will-power, a successful trial to walk with cruthches all the way from Katra to Vaishnodevi a distance of 15 Kms was tried in September 1989. The feeling of success in the mission goes long way in creating sense of pride which keeps tension away.

8. **Sever your attachment :** Many of the problems that we have, can be imaginatively solved by severing with a thing. We ourselves create attachment with so many worldly things and on non-achievement of the thing we ourselves feel bad, i.e., most of the problems that we solve within the circumstances of desire are self-generated by us.

   Once we remove that curtain, we can have insight of a thing. The change of attitude by severing relationship with his leg by saying, "I am alright, it is the bad luck of leg which is suffering". Now by shifting this severing concept from inner self to a particular part of body, one can still enjoy more by calling your own part of body as something which is foreign to self.

9. **Live in reality :** Understand a thing, come to reality, reduce gap between your expectation and reality to reduce tension. People love you not because you are good but also on account of how far you can solve their selfish interests.

   Identification of true caring friends took long time because I was always under wrong impression that doing good always begets a good. There is no doubt that "Good begets good" but if you take in relative sense that all those with whom you exchange pleasantry are your real friends is wrong. It is necessary to distinguish those who are attracted towards you because you are good in general sense. Only from that group we can expect the role of true friendship. As far as the other group who are attracted towards you because you can solve their selfish interest and not because you are good in general. Once this distinction is understood you are less likely to be entrapped in tension at a time when you are in real trouble. The principle that can be derived from this situation is that many problems of tension occur due to lack of knowledge. Once we start realising the truth, there is likely to be less gap between expectation and reality and hence we are less likely to be affected by tension. More the gap we keep between reality and expectation, we are likely to be affected by increased tension.

10. **Artificiality createas tension, accept the reality:** It is said "God loves you for what you are and not for what you should be". The friendship can subsist longer if both the persons involved accept the reality of the counterpart. A friendship based on artificiality cannot subsist for long.

A clear distinction should be made when we are not capable of realising the goal and hence never fix unrealistic target. This faulty type of target fixation creates artificial picture before the people around you or this may be due to ego problem. This generated artificiality by our own self can be the cause of tension.

Obviously, this became clear while waiting in queue meant for getting handicapped certificate. The inner heart was not accepting the reality of being labelled and called 'handicapped'. To satisfy inner heart, the author recollects his asking for a disability certificate in place of 'handicapped certificate'. This was giving different colour to problem. So, it is necessary to accept fact. Just by giving colour to the satisfying the fact can't be changed, that must be realised.

11. **Strong will-power solves problems of tension :** Don't take outside help of sympathy as a solution. Sympathy from other people makes you accept the situation. Sympathy should not come in your way as it dampens motivation.

Sympathy may resolve the problem temporarily. It may be necessary to make you not fall in the depression-trap in the case of negative solution. One can't have sympathy from every one around his. It must be understood that we should try to become more and more efficient and proficient in different field to make ourselves survive. "The fittest alone will survive" is the slogan. Don't accept the defeat. It is relevant to increase will power. When one becomes determined with strong will, many problems that are created by tension are not likely to take birth or the influence of them can be minimised to a good extent.

12. **Good time and bad time are two sides of same coin :** It must be understood that the concept of sadness must be understood for the enjoyment of happy moments. Down is bound to come after every night every hill has a valley, every sea has a shore, spring is bound to come after every autum.

Publishers' Note

A sad note to share with our readers! Navin successfully struggled for eight years to save his left leg but finally he had to get it amputed when this book was under publication. I wish the authors good health.

Satish Jain

2

THE SPECTRUM OF TENSION

Tension is a term which psychologists have borrowed from physics. It is physiological (bio-chemical) change resulting from an overloading force on the system. Every physiological change is likely to produce corresponding psychological change and conversely every psychological change may lead to physiological change.

Before we get into the term tension and explain the ways and means to get rid of it, it is important to understand the nature of stress. Stress is a global term and tension is simply one form of stress. The word stress comes from the latin word **stringere,** which means "to draw tight". Stress is one's physical, mental and chemical response to things that frighten, excite, confuse, endanger or irritate. Stress varies on a continuum from Eustress or Neustress and finally to Distress. When the stress is unfavourable and potentially disease producing, it is labelled as distress or tension. When an individual is able to maintain steady internal state as a stress response, it is known as neustress. If stress response is favourable and results in improvement in physical and mental functioning, it is called eustress. The effect of stress is dependent on the type of stressors and weight that an individual attaches to the stressors while reacting. To place this reaction in mathematical formula, S-O-R (Stress Organism - Response) can be defined as :

$$R = f (S.O.)$$

where,   R is response to stressful situation

S - Stressors

O - Organism that is being stimulated

f - Function of

The response is thus dependent on type of stressor and how an individual, who is involved, reacts to a particular situation. Before one proceeds further, it is necessary to understand the term 'Stressor". Stressor is the agent or demand that evokes a patterned response, it is that which causes stress.

It must be understood that there is need to maintain balance of body, mind and spirit. There is need to find a way between the extremes of hypo and hyper tension and both are bad for an individual. One can have hypo-stress by having physical immobility, boredom and sensory deprivation.

Selye (1979) suggests that all organisms go through a General Adaptation Syndrome (GAS) which passes through three stages –

(a) Alarm reaction which is comprised of shock phase (the initial and immediate reaction to a noxious agent) and counter shock phase, a mobilisation of defence phases in which the adrenal cortex becomes further enlarged and secretes more costicoid hormones.

(b) Stage of resistance which involves adapting to the stressror stimulus but decreasing one's ability to cope with subsequent stimulus.

(c) Stage of exhaustion which follows a period of prolonged or severe adaptation.

Tension imposes demand on the body for its proper adaptation. If it is not handled carefully, it may cause inbreeding of various diseases in the body. Every disease in turn causes certain amount of tension as it demands need for adaptation. The effects of tension may be cured by various therapies such as shock therapy, physical therapy, occupational therapy etc. The effects of tension are damaging when they go beyond the adaptability level. Tension effects the weakest limb of the body which is manifested in the form of various diseases of nervous system, gastrointestinal tract, heart problem and the like.

There is need to maintain balance of mind. Some people experience grief which directs their psychic energy inward against their own natural body defences. Different persons' respond to a particular tension provoking situation differently:

There is need to develop a balanced state of mind to convert the stress responses into beneficial effects. Though the cause of tension can be failure, it should be taken as a stepping stone for success. Tension can also be due to mishaps. Mishaps are like knives that either serve us or cut us. It is necessary to evaluate one's performance, as success is never final and failure is never fatal, it is the courage that counts.

Human body reacts both mentally and physically in stressful situations which leads to 'flight or fight' responses. Psychoneuro-immunologists believe that stress affects people infected with Human Immunological deficiency Virus (HIV) which develops AIDS and even shorten length of their survival. Latest studies reported at American Association for Advancement of Science Convention at San Fransisco held in January 1990 have indicated that stress can be linked with various illnesses especially those caused by latent viruses e.g. stress can activate the herpes viruses which may lie dormant in the body for years.

Tension affects the whole body, it is merely a question as to which part breaks first. The great enemy of human health is not the occasional crisis or dangerous situation but it is the prolonged unrelieved state of worry, anxiety and arousal that people experience and can't escape.

BODY PARTS AND THEIR FUNCTIONING

The negative effects on different parts of body due to tension can be better understood if one understands the various functions of these parts.

1. Heart
   (a) Regulates circulation of blood.

(b) Controls mental activity.

(c) Couples with the blood vessels.

(d) Couples with the small intestines.

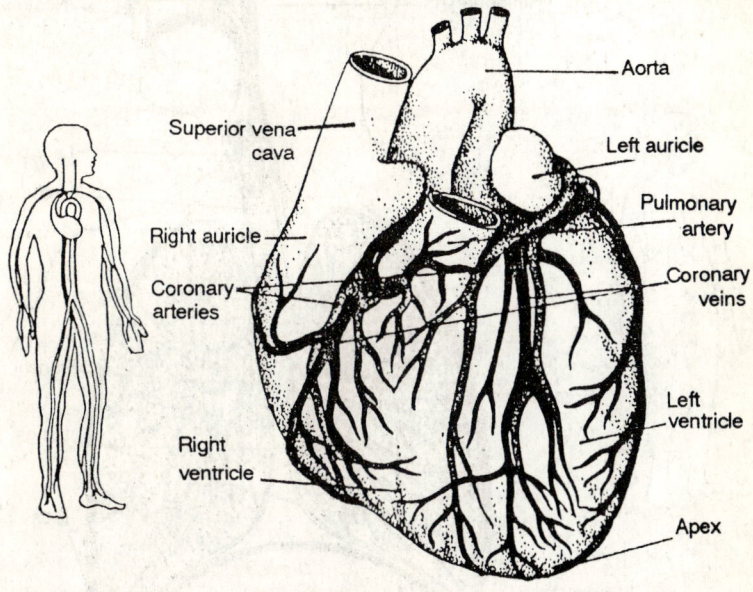

Fig. 2.1 : Circulatory system and heart.

2. Lungs

(a) Regulate respiration.

(b) All blood travels to the lungs and then circulates.

(c) Govern the skin and body hair.

(d) Couple with large intestines.

3. Spleen

(a) Regulates digestion.

(b) Controls water metabolism.

(c) Controls the circulation of the blood.

(d) Governs muscles (Soft tissues) and the four extremities (limbs).

(e) Supplies nutrition to the tongue and the lips.

(f) Spleen couples with the stomach.

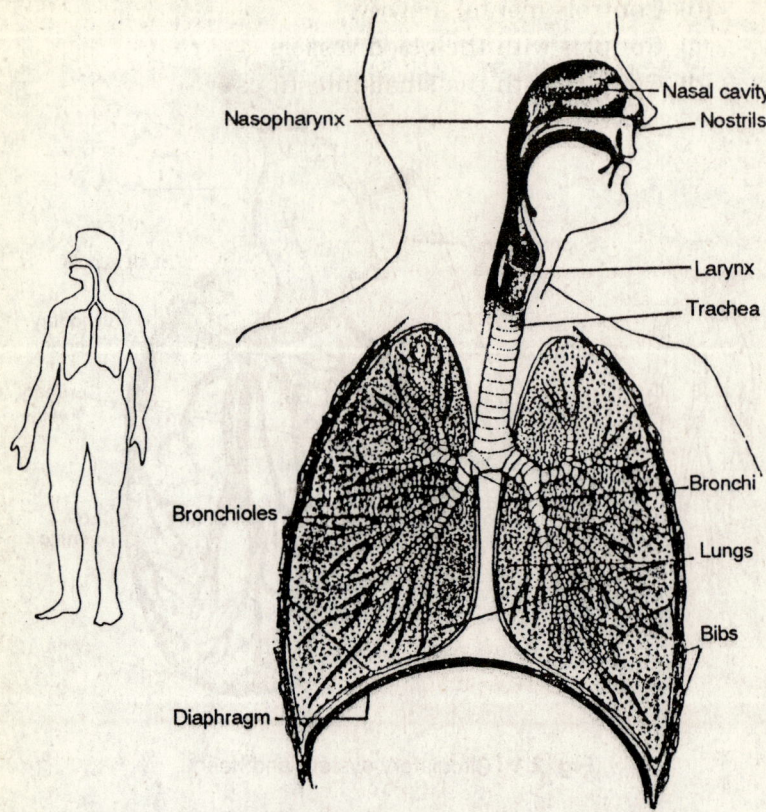

Fig. 2.2 : Respiratory system & lungs.

4. Liver

(a) Stores and regulates the blood.

(b) Secretes bile.

(c) Governs the tendons and endocrines.

(d) It transports blood, bile and endocrines.

(e) Couples with the Gall bladder.

5. Kidneys

(a) Regulate bone growth and teeth development.

(b) Govern bones, cartilage and head hair.

(c) Generate vital essences.

(d) Promote new life.

(e) Couple with the urinary bladder.

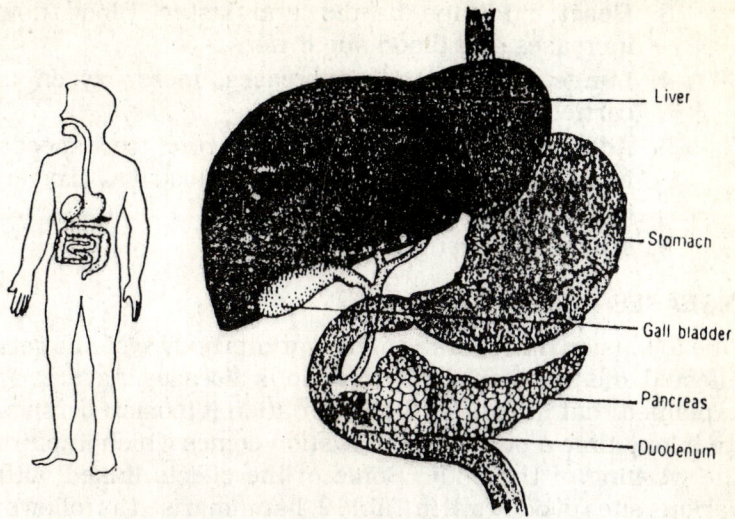

Fig. 2.3 : Digestive system and spleen & liver.

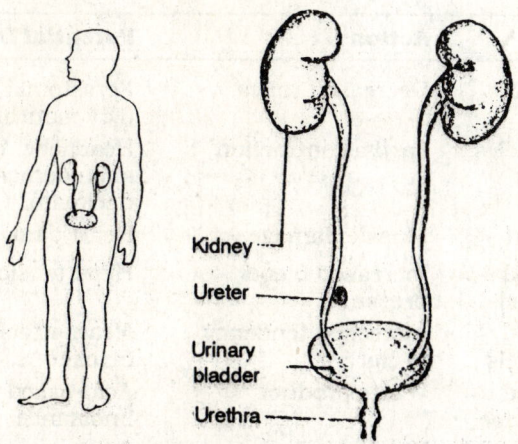

Fig. 2.4 : Excretery system and kidneys.

The working of all these parts gets affected during tension and following effects can be noticed :

1. **Brain :** Sympathetic nerves and pituitary gland get stimulated.

2. **Spinal cord :** Sympathetic and parasympathetic nerves stimulate organs.

3. **Heart :** Pumps harder and faster, Blood flow increases and blood sugar rises.
4. **Lungs :** Respiration increases, more oxygen is carried.
5. **Adrenal Glands :** Andrenaline is produced, speeds heart rate, respiration, improves blood flow, oxygen consumption, muscle strength.
6. **Muscles :** Strength increases.

DISEASES – Due to Tension

Due to tension, functioning of the various body systems gets affected and that gives birth to various diseases. As already explained that in fight or flight' situation if tension persists for a long time a period of exhaustion comes which impairs the working of the body. Some of the effects linked with various sites of body are in Table 2.1 summarised as follows:

Table 2.1 : Effects Linked with Body Sites.

	Site	Action	Potential Disease
1.	Mouth	Decreased saliva	Xerostomia (Dry mouth)
2.	Muscles	Partial contraction	Headache, backache, shoulderache, neckpain
3.	Heart	Muscle damage	Heart damage
4.	Blood vessels	Increased blood pressure	Hypertension
5.	Blood vessels	Increased tendency to clot	Heart attack or Stroke
6.	Blood Lactage	Waste product	Acid-based imbalance
7.	Uric acid	Waste product	Gout
8.	Lungs	Increased breathing rates, vascular change	Hyper ventilation, impaired breathing
9.	Lungs	Excessive Dilation	Impaired breathing
10.	Liver	Excessive Glucose	Diabetes
11.	Skin	Vasoconstriction	Pallor

Untoward musculoskeleton reactions and physio-pathological disorders and emotional disturbance may arise due to stress. The reason is constant bombardment of cerebral control centres by proprioceptive impulses originating in tense muscles. This hyperarousal may result in :

   (i)   Flushing
  (ii)   Sweating
 (iii)   Chilling
  (iv)   Upset stomach
   (v)   Constipation
  (vi)   Diarrhea
 (vii)   Palpitation
(viii)   Blurred vision
  (ix)   Dry mouth
   (x)   Wet hands and feet.

Blood Pressure

With every contraction and relaxation of heart, there is a certain degree of pressure on the walls of the blood vessels and this is called blood pressure. Tension directly affects the blood pressure in a person. Severity of hypertension is determined more by the diastolic pressure (lower) as compared to systolic pressure (upper) as greater fluctuation comes in upper pressure. During stress thyrotropic hormone (T.T.H.) is released, it goes to thyroid gland and causes the release of thyroxine and other thyroid hormones. Hypothalamus activates the posterior pituitary gland resulting in release of Vasopressin hormone which acts on arteries causing them to contract, Thus raising the blood pressure.

The symptoms that are developed due to hypertension leading to imbalance in blood pressure are as follows :

   (a)   Heaviness of head
   (b)   Breathlessness on mild physical exertion
   (c)   Lack of concentration at work
   (d)   Impaired vision
   (e)   Disturbed sleep
   (f)   Feeling of generalised heaviness of body

The various bad implications of tension which result due to severity of blood pressure, lead to various silent diseases and if the same is not cured, it results in :

   (a)   Strokes

    (b) Heart attacks

    (c) Angina

    (d) Blindness

    (e) Kidney failure.

Most of the drugs prescribed for treatment of high blood pressure have side effects. Some of the drugs for curing high blood pressure result in increase in sugar in blood, uric acid, blood lipids. Some medicines lead the subject to fatigue, depression, and even impaired sex life.

Effects on Digestive System

Tension affects the working of digestive system. Before one understands the negative effects, it is necessary to understand the role of digestive system in the body. The object of digestion is to convert the food into a fluid state that is capable of being absorbed by the blood. The blood in turn supplies oxygen to various organs of the body, removes

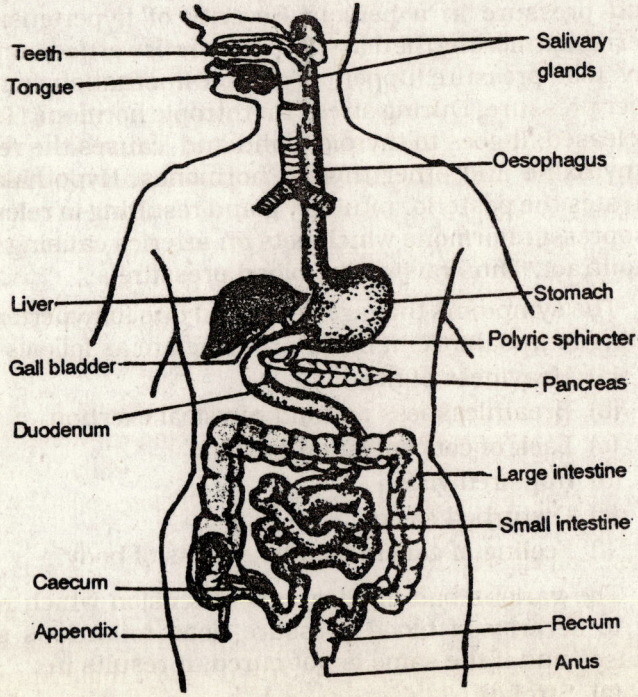

Fig. 2.5 : Indicating human digestive system.

waste of the body and produces digestive juices. Digestive system basically consists of 31 feet long tube called Alimentary canal. The six organs which absorb food and extract the waste are as follows :

(a) **Stomach** : The digestion, ingestion and transportation of food and water (fluids) is done by the stomach.

(b) **Small Intestine** : It separates the essence from the waste of food and transports the latter to the large intestine.

(c) **Large Intestine** : It extracts the wastes.

(d) **Gall Bladder** : It stores biles, controls mental activities, maintains integrity of all muscles.

(e) **Urinary Bladder** : It is a part of body situated in the front part of the pelvic cavity, which acts as a reservoir of urine.

(f) **Sandiod Bladder** : It controls the homeostasis of the body.

How Digestion Suffers in Tension

Under tension a person's muscle tone quickly increases, making muscular action more immediate and more efficient. The liver immediately begins working to convert its stored **glycogen** into **glucose**, which the brain and muscles need in greater supply. The breathing becomes more rapid and intense, increasing the supply of oxygen into the blood. The heart pumps more rapidly and intensively sending an abundant supply of blood to those portions of the body which need it. The distribution of the blood throughout the body is radically changed, according to a suddenly revised system of priority. The plentiful supply of blood into one's stomach and intestines is quickly reduced in favour of higher priority needs. This is one reason why digestion suffers in prolonged stress.

Effects on Reproductive System

The general effects of the tension are to diminish the overall functioning of the male sex apparatus. Prolonged stress sharply decreases the level of the primary male hormone, testosterone, which directly influences the sex drive. Stress slows down, the production of sperm cells in the male (Kenneth Lammott, 1975). In females, during prolonged stress, progesterone, the principal female hormone, diminishes sharply. Reduction in progesterone can cause menstrual irregularities.

Infection-Bearing Capacity Decreases

Cortisol and other similar hormones have many actions which allow the body to deal adaptively with stressors for long periods of time during the stage of resistance. It is harmful for the body to remain in high levels of tension which require more corticol hormones. Cortisol promotes the formation of glucose (blood sugar), by breaking down fats and proteins. In shortrun, this increased use of protein may be serious because proteins are needed in the manufacturing of new cells. White blood cells which are crucial for fighting infection have a short life and must be continuously replaced. If the proteins need to make new cells are used for fuel then the ability of the body to fight the infection decreases.

Other Changes in Tension

Researchers have observed that following changes take place when a person is tense :

(a) Hearing becomes acute.

(b) Vision becomes more sensitive – pupil of eyes dilate which makes vision more sensitive.

(c) Blood Clotting – Clotting agent in blood streams increases which can lead to minor malfunctioning to total paralysis.

(d) Skin Resistance – It has been observed that during tension, there are changes in electrical resistance of the skin. During tension normally the skin's surface temperature goes down.

3

THOUGHT PROCESS :
ROOT OF TENSION

HUMAN MIND

To understand the various facets of 'Tension', it is necessary to understand 'Human mind', the origin of thought processes. All the human beings have structurally the same brain but its functioning varies. The functioning determines success or failure, reward or punishment, rejection or honour of an individual. Human mind in physiological terms, is called brain which weighs approximately three pounds in an average adult human being. Mind controls, governs and guides the activities of the entire body system which in turn controls the heart beats, rate of respiration, the generative parts, the various glands and their secretions.

A person is what his mind is. Human mind is restless by nature and it creates a restless world around itself. The more it gets, the more it craves for. The vicious circle of endless desires intoxicate it and gradually it gives way to feelings of jealousy, pride and ambition and other demonic traits like enmity and egoism. Mind is a multi-level phenomenon and there are certain areas of mind which cannot be reached by conscious ego of the individual. It may not be an exaggeration to say that each person is a mystery unto himself. Tension in mind affects temperament of a person and ungoverned temper affects the whole system of a human being including all organs, limbs and senses.

The Sankhya School of Indian Philosophy believes that the entire world including human being is a manifestation of male prakriti, which is constitute of (a) Sattwa, (b) Rajas and (c) Tamas Gunas. Human body is a synthesis of Sattwa, Rajas and Tamas. **Sattwa** is indicator of happiness, virtue and knowledege. **Rajas** leads to action which rouses attachment and vision of multiplicity. **Tamas** casts a veil of ignorance over one's mind and one falls asleep spiritually.

The combinations of these gunas determine the quality of a person in terms of **sukh, dukh** and **moha. Sukh** in terms of sincerity, respect, forbearance, kindness are sattwa qualities. **Dukh** in terms of spite, anger and other immoral emotions are Rajas qualities. **Moha** in terms of fear, scepticism, crookedness represent Tamas qualities. These three gunas are, therefore, regarded primarily as feelings which hold within themselves the germs of differences and diversities. The identical nature of mind is explained well by Yogic concept of Sahasra and Muladhara. In yoga, the human brain is a mass of tissues, whose structure, composition, shape and form resemble the shape and form of a lotus flower. The lotus has thousands of petals which are symbolized in the brain by a series of folds of ridges called a convolution of gunas. Like the lotus flower the brain is attached to its stem which is called the Spinal cord. Further as lotus stem is rooted in the ground from which it receives nourishment, energy or life, so also the brain-stem (the spinal cord) is rooted in the Muladhara which is physiologically termed as Sacrum. According to the Yogic concept the source of all energy is Muladhara which acts like the root by serving as the source of energy, power and life to the lotus flower.

The other similarity of the brain and lotus flower is as follows :

Lotus grows in water and its stem is vertical in shape from the root upto the surface of water where it holds the flower. The spinal cord is also vertical from Muladhara upto the base of the brain. As lotus flower is on the top of its stem so is the Sahasra (the brain) on the top its stem (the spine) and they are surrounded by a fluid known as cerebrospinal fluid. **Muladhara** is a Sanskrit word consisting of **Mula** which means the root and **Adhara** which means the foundation or the base. **Muladhara** is that part of porenium, where the anus and the genitals meet. In yogic concepts reproductive glands have been regarded as sources of energy. The mental level disparity exists from a person to person because of differences of knowledge motivation values, interests, training disciplinary habits, way of life and inherent power. The composition and qualities of the mind at the time of birth are the same in all persons, but they start differentiating and varying due to the environment in which they are brought up.

4

TENSION :
ANATOMY AND PHYSIOLOGY

A recession is a period in which one tightens one's belt, depression is a time when one has no belt to tighten and it is tension period when one has no trousers to hold. The French blame their liver for all their ills, the Indians blame their stars, while Americans attribute everything to stress. Researchers have lent respectability to the American notion by linking central nervous system to the activity of immune system.

Nervous system consists of nerves, brain and spinal cord. It controls the working of various organs of the body. Studies by Psycho-physiologists show that the bodily changes, that occur during tension, are produced by autonomic nervous system which is a part of peripheral nervous system. The autonomic nervous system physiologically consists of many nerves leading from brain and spinal cord to smooth muscle of various organs of the body, to the heart, to certain glands and to the blood vessels which serve both the interior and the exterior parts of the body. The autonomic nervous system, from functioning point of view, consists of two parts –

(a) Sympathetic nervous system, and

(b) Para-sympathetic nervous system

Sympathetic nervous system is active during aroused state and para-sympathetic system is active in calm and relaxed state. There is need to maintain a balance of sympathetic and para-sympathetic nervous system activities to get optimum result. The control and regulation of the functioning of internal organs is the work of para-sympathetic nerves. In case of stress, sympathetic nerves take over and release a chemical substance called **adrenaline** at their nerve ends and send to different organs of the body. The purpose of adrinaline is to prepare the body to fight stress. From neurological point of view, when one is chronically tense one loses the ability to mobilise one's para-sympathetic system. If the gap between aroused state and calm state increases, one becomes tense. The optimum level of result can be obtained when the gap between the functioning of the two remains within the permissible limit. When one adopts relaxation technique, one's capacity to match with aroused state of affair increases. This can be understood from Fig. 4.1.

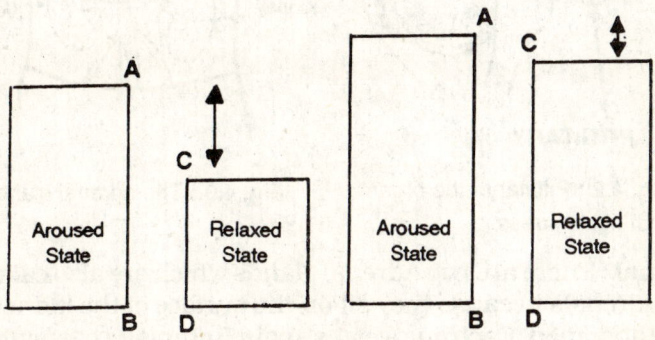

Fig. 4.1

Both diagrams show permissible arousal state, because the gap between AB and CD remains within permissible limit. When the imbalance occurs there is need to :

1. Reduce arousal state activities or
2. Increase relaxed state activities.

THE CHEMISTRY OF TENSION

External stimuli from environment are perceived by cerebral cortex of the brain. This information is passed to hypothala-mus, which in turn passes information on to the pituitary gland which controls the release of all the hormones for the purpose of taking up different activities.

Pituitary : This gland lies in underface of the brain at the base of the skull. Its size is about the size of a pea and weighs about half a gram. Pituitary has two parts viz. : (a) Anterior lobe (b) Posterior lobe. The former produces about ten hormones and the latter produces about two hormones. Pituitary gland controls the activities of the whole body by affecting thyroid, the adrenals, sex glands etc.

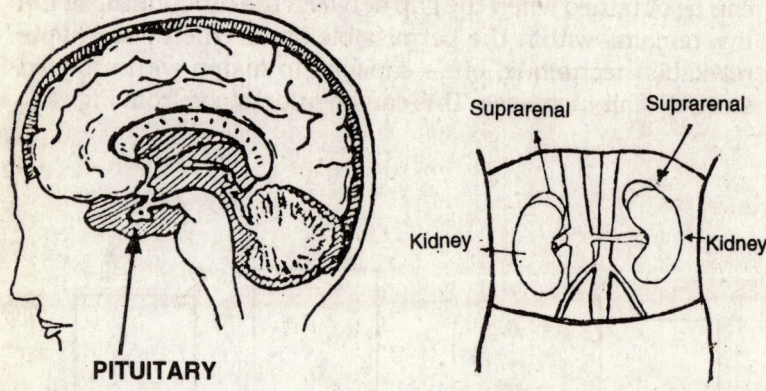

Fig. 4.2 : Pituitary - the organ that fights stress.

Fig. 4.3 : The adrenal glands.

Adrenal : There are two Adrenal glands which are also called supradrenals because they sit on the surface of the kidneys in the abdomen. Each one weighs about 5 grams, is triangular in shape and is about the size of the last phalanx of the thumb. The inner core of this is called medulla and the outer portion is called cortex. The release of hormones from this gland is small in quantity but is very powerful. The two important hormones that are released by the medulla of the Adrenal after receiving impulses from Hypothalamus which in turn receives message from Cerebral cortex which initially senses the stress. The two harmones released in the blood stream are :

(a) Adrenaline

(b) Nordrenaline.

The release of these hormones in the blood, make the liver to release more glucose (source of energy) and constrict capillaries in the skin which make it look pale and the blood of the skin gets diverted to the muscle and the internal organs. The heart rate increases, the arteries constrict and as a result the blood pressure rises. The digestion system gets stopped because in the in-built system this is not considered important. Clotting time of blood is lessened and bleeding stops from the wound.

To nullify the bad effect of tension, impulses from the Hypothalamus stimulate the Pituitary gland to release another hormone called ACTH (Andreno Corticotrophic Hormone). This hormone acts upon the cortex of the adrenals and make it release its hormone in the blood. The purpose of the release of these hormones is to bring normal state in the body by bringing down the raised blood pressure by dilating the blood vessels. The complex in-built system equips the individual to handle the stressful situation but prolonged period of tension leads to overburdening of the system. This becomes starting point of diseases like stomach ulceration, heart trouble, and high blood pressure.

5

MEDIATORS OF TENSION

INTRODUCTION

Charles Bukowski, a poet, has written : "It is not the large things that send a man to the mad house ...... no, it's the continuing series of small tragedies that send a man to the mad house." We all live in a world of stress and strain. As the complexities of living increase, human life tends to become tense. According to the American Academy of Family Physicians, two-third of the patients visiting the family doctors suffer from emotional disturbances and show tension-related symptoms.

Mediators of tension lie either in the environment or in the individual as tension is a particular kind of commerce between a person and his surroundings. There are two points of view, one is environmentalistic and the other is organismic. The former believes that the cause of tension lies only in the environment whereas the latter solely attributes tension to individual's personality make-up. Researches confirm that both the environment and the personality are crucial factors in deciding the level of tension. The level of tension is an interaction of person with his environment e.g. a person may be tense because external demand seems very taxing and sources for managing it are weak, it may be due to a weak demand that nevertheless appears stronger than the available resources for managing it. While describing organismic point of view, one should keep individual's biological, psychological characteristics in mind. Reaction of individuals, to the same environmental events, varies in quality, intensity and duration e.g. the effect of noise may create irritation in one person's mind but the other person may be comfortable.

PSYCHOLOGICAL MEDIATORS

The outcome of stressful transaction depends upon types of tension-provoking episodes and their perceived importance. Every individual has his own way of evaluating a situation. One always reacts not only to a situation but the way a situation is perceived specially in relation to one's ability to cope with it. One might meet an individual undergoing a severe tension but on analysing the cause that has produced tension after discussing with another person, one may conclude the causes are not strong enough to produce high level of tension.

1. Personality Traits

To understand the role of individual personality traits as mediators of tension, it is important to understand the traits. Four of these are listed below :

(i) **Hardiness** : People with more hardiness have stronger commitment to self and have a sense of meaningfulness. They feel they can manage things according to their desires. They have an ability to feel deeply involved in or committed to an activity of their life. They perceive tension provoking situations as challenging. These people are cognitively flexible which allows them to integrate and effectively appraise the threat of new situations. When people with higher degree of hardiness experience high degree of tension due to personality structure, chances of their falling ill are rare than those with lower level of hardiness, as the former can control/ influence the events of their experience and they very seldom undergo high tension state.

(ii) **Optimism Vs. Pessimism :** The individuals who are pessimistic in life perceive a tension provoking situation as potentially damaging or threatening to survival. On the contrary, an optimistic individual will perceive the same situation as challenging.

(iii) **Stress Tolerance :** The severity of a given stress depends on resources for withstanding tension in general and that stress in particular. If a person is marginally adjusted, (i.e. not easily adjusted) the slightest tension may be highly damaging. Stress tolerance refers to one's ability to withstand stress without having integrated functioning impaired seriously. Both biologically and psychologically, people vary to a great extent in vulnerability to tension. Sometimes, earlier traumatic experiences leave an individual particularly vulnerable to that kind of tension.

(iv) **Locus of Control :** Control is generalised belief of an individual regarding the extent to which one can control the outcome of self and environment. There are two kinds of people. First are the internally controlled persons and the other are the externally controlled persons. Internally controlled persons are confident of self in dealing with the happenings of life, whereas externally controlled persons feel the things surrounding them are controlled by other powerful persons i.e. A wife can feel most of the things which concern her, are decided by her husband. At a work place, it can be the boss or a colleague. Locus of control has been found by Lefcourt (1984) to act as a mediator of the outcome of stressful life events. People who have more perceived control, deal with tension provoking situations with courage and confidence, whereas the externally controlled people perceive such situations as threatening to life.

2. Environmental Factors

Lack of personal and materialistic external support makes a given tension more severe and weaken an individual's capacity to cope with it. A divorce or a death of one's mate is more stressful if one is still surrounded by people who care. So this shows that it is not only the tension provoking episode or the individual traits which decide the intensity of tension but also the environmental factors, in which the episode takes place.

3. Perceptual Factors

Any situation which one perceives as threatening is much more stressful than the one that is perceived as presenting a difficult but manageable problem. Tension provoking situations, which are potentially damaging or threatening to survival carry a high degree of tension e.g. being given a diagnosis of a terminal disease or having a limb amputated. Similarly, a situation that threatens the adequacy of desires incompatible with one's self concept and self ideas, that questions the worth of self, also creates a very high degree of tension.

OTHER MEDIATORS

Many people believe that the solution of tension lies in excitements and intoxicants. In this chapter, an introduction has been given to such thrilling and excitement creating factors and their scientifically proved effects have been deliberated upon.

Vivid descriptions of the diseases produced due to tension have been scientifically explained. Tension acts like a silent killer, the universal rise in tension in day to day life and its bad effects have emphasised the need to study tension and its curative and preventive aspects.

1. Diet

The type of food one takes has a great bearing on determining one's competence to deal with situations which are tension provoking. Basically all foods can be classified as :

(a) Energy yielding foods : These are rich in carbohydrates and fats (like sugar, curds etc.)

(b) Body building foods : These foods are rich in proteins (e.g. milk, pulse etc.)

(c) Protective foods : These foods are rich in proteins, minerals and vitamins (e.g. milk, egg. green vegetables etc.)

As metabolic or dietary deficiency can cause an anxious state viz. tension, it is necessary to understand the role of carbohydrates, proteins, fats, vitamins and minerals. The requirement of these different things varies from person to person on the basis of sex and level of physical activity. Under these important heads of diet the following three significant viewpoints are worth considering.

(a) Scientific view point
(b) Nature cure view point
(c) Philosophical view point

(a) SCIENTIFIC VIEW POINT

Food is digested and then absorbed through the process of oxidation. Oxidation is a controlled process during which energy is released in a number of steps rather than in an instantaneous combustion.

Proteins help in the process of digestion. Proteins are broken into acids and circulated out of the body via the liver. Human body uses very little proteins for energy except as a last resort in a situation of starving or getting too little carbohydrate.

Fats too travel through liver and body cells. To convert fat into energy, oxygen is needed whereas there is no need in case of carbohydrates. First Carbohydrates are converted into energy unlike fats which are used when carbohydrates are not available. Fats provide cushions to vital organs and they supply vitamins A, B, E and K. Carbohydrates provide energy at first instance as they adopt digestive track. Their first action starts through saliva and ends in small intestine. The small intestine breaks them into simple sugars and these are all converted into glucose by the liver. Glucose is sent to heart for circulation throughout the body. Ideal food with all the three organic components, is available in form of milk, vegetables, fruits, cereals and meat. Salt plays an important role for hypertensive patients. Research studies show that high intake of sodium salt leads to high blood pressure whereas potassium salt has been found to help in reducing high blood pressure.

Acid Forming Food vs. Alkali Forming Food

It has been established that chemical imbalance comes in body when there exists an excess percentage of acid forming food as compared to alkali forming food. It has been considered that 80% alkali forming food and 20% acid forming food is ideal to create chemical balance in body. Raw salads, juices, raw vegetables etc. come in the category of alkali forming food whereas fried things, rice, custard etc. come in the category of acid forming food.

Cooked vs. Uncooked Food

There are certain foods, which when taken in raw form, carry more nutritive value. There are certain foods which should be taken in cooked form to make them digestible like raw fish, meat, potatoes etc. Cooking of certain foods is necessary to kill micro-organisms which would otherwise be harmful to our system.

Vegetarian vs. Non-vegetarian Food

It has been established through studies that high blood pressure on the whole has been found less in vegetarian food group as compared to non-vegetarian group. In terms of analysis of studies, non-vegetarians are more prone to high blood pressure due to :

(a) more polyunsaturated fats

(b) easy digestibility of dietary fibres in vegetable food

(c) presence of high levels of potassium in vegetable diet

It has been scientifically established that alpha activity is induced more by vegetable meals than by non vegetable ones. A vegetarian diet reduces acidity. In terms of the results of Mayo clinic in U.S.A., the relationship between vitamin B deprivation and behavioural problems have been conclusively proved. Deficiency of vitamin B or thiamine can increase the production of adrenaline in the body. Adrenaline promotes the 'fight or flight' syndrome which is not the normal behaviour, making the individual more irritable, quarrelsome, non-cooperative and even depressed. The research has concluded that restoration of vitamin B to the diet of the volunteers soon made them cheerful and physically better. The appalling increase in juvenile delinquency and adult crimes can be due to the increased use of refined carbohydrates and chemicals added to processed food. Latest studies have proved that brain is vulnerable to nutritional fluctuations. The biochemistry and function of brain gets affected with the alteration of nearly a dozen specific nutrients.

Vitamin B plays a vital role in the functioning of body. Brain needs glucose, which is being supplied by vitamin B for its efficient use. Deficiency of this creates nutritional imbalance leading to emotional imbalance which is manifested by the body through fatigue, depression, irritation, nervousness, insomnia etc. The psychiatric and neurological symptoms like depression, nervousness, fatigue etc. can be cured by increasing the intake of thiamine, riboflavine, folate, potassium, iron, ponotothenate, B6, B12. Iron helps to form haemoglobin, a substance in red cells (RBC) which carries oxygen from lungs to the rest of the body. Deficiency of iron results in less supply of oxygen to various tissues and this leads to the feeling of fatigue. This results in shortage of breath, increase in heart beat which ultimately leads to a run down feeling. Calcium is available in yoghurt, skimmed milk and swiss cheese etc. 99% of our body's calcium is present in the bones and teeth. The one per cent which is present in the soft tissues and blood plays important role to create its impact on the nerves. Calcium shortage affects the emotional balance which results in irritability, tense disposition, insomnia, loss of memory etc.

Magnesium is available in soyabean, almonds etc. It is a very natural sedative which creates calming effects in the body. Shortage of this results in anxiety, insomnia and depression.

(b) NATURE CURE VIEW POINT

Nature cure approach evaluates the role of food in terms of vital power. It is important to remember that food is not complete unless and until it gets absorbed and assimilated in the inner system of body. If the food remains unassimilated due to malfunctioning of the system then unassimilated food becomes the seed of disease.

Food is taken by us either by licking, sucking, chewing or by way of sipping. Food except in body building stage, can tax the vital power. Its purpose is only to replace waste cells. In modern life, due to the changing styles of living, it can be said that the greatest and most culpable waste of power takes place through eating. Thus vital power can be saved by reducing this waste to a bare minimum.

After an average quantity of meal all the vital energies are called up from elsewhere and yoked to the task of food disposal. First the energy is drawn away from the legs and the man wants to sit. Then it is also withdrawn from the upper muscles and the individual is unable to sit upright, he wants to lean or lie down and sleep for an hour or more.

As the greatest and most culpable waste of power takes place through eating, the greatest and most profitable economies of vital power are thus possible by stopping this waste or by reducing it to a minimum

(c) PHILOSOPHICAL VIEW POINT

The philosophical view emphasises the role of food in determining the nature of a person. The Bhagavat Gita has classified various types of food in terms of three gunas mentioned earlier i.e. Sattwa, Rajas and Tamas. Food habits help in one's efforts to preserve Sattwa qualities. Sattwa guna qualities lead to clarity and mental serenity. They develop when we take things which promote life, vitality, health, joy and cheerfulness. Rajas gunas make a person active and energetic, tense and wilful. All these are cultivated though foods which are harsh, salty, bitter, sour, hot, pungent or burn producing Tamas qualities obstruct and counteract the tendency of Rajas to work and Satwa to reveal. Tamas gunas cultivate when we take foods which are non-consamable, tasteless, unclean, stale etc.

Vedanta emphasised that the kind of food one takes has its effect in determining the nature of the person. As per this view, non-vegetarian food distracts concentration of power which is most needed for a student of religion and hence must be avoided by those who wish to attain higher order of spiritualism. Satvic food has been emphsised by ISKCON and Brahma Kumaries (Raja yoga). As per them meat, alcohol, tobacco, spicy, passion inducing foods, onions and garlic must be avoided.

All the philosophical approaches have accepted the fact that the kind of food that one eats, creates the impact which in total determines one's nature. After alcohol consumption a person is bound to become intoxicated. If a person takes opium the effect of the same will control that person. So each type of food produces different types of effects that affect the nature of a person.

2. Fasting

Fasting plays an important role in revitalising the various organs of the body. Fasting or starvation produces mental stimulation, the brain becomes more excited and is in a better position to cope with the problems in a better way. It starts working faster and more accurately with less sense of fatigue. Fasting has been used as an important tool for purification of body and mind. The role of fasting has been duly recognised by Gandhiji in his preachings.

The basic principle behind fasting is that during the fast the body adjusts itself vigorously between a state of disease and a state of high level of health and that too in a short period of time. In fasting, energy gets diverted from external muscles to most urgent work on hand, which is to do internal cleaning of the body. This shifting of energy makes the person on fast feel weak. Even energy is diverted from the brain which does intellectual work for the purpose of purification of body. When the energy is withdrawn from stomach and small intestine, digestive juices become less and as such no digestion takes place and this leads to lack of appetite. In fasting consumption of condiments, spices and salts goes down and thus the withdrawal system makes the individual realise the factual position of the weakness of the body. Once this internal cleaning process is done, vital energy is used for active working of different organs of the body. Fasting goes a long way in improving the health in real sense and this process raises the competence of the individual to deal with stressful situation.

3. Caffeine

The effect of caffeines can be rightly observed in the conversation between two friends, "We used to sit up all night discussing nation's problems over cigarettes and coffee. Now our problem is cigarettes and coffee."

In modern life, use of stimulants/stimulators has increased in our food and drink items. Excessive use of stimulators in one's day-to-day life directly taxes one's energy. It creates situations of emergency. These stimulators only tax existing energy and have bad effects on body system even if occasionally used.

Caffeine is present in coffee, tea, certain soft drinks and in some proprietary medication. The excessive use of the products containing caffeine results in stimulation of the nervous system. Stimulation through caffeine leads to weakness of nerves. The caffeine stimulates the flow of gastric juices. This repeated stimulation weakens the ability of the systems to secrete the digestive juices. Caffeine affects the heart by causing it to beat irregularly. Stimulation makes the heart beat rate faster.

James S.M. Closter has stated in his book Nutrition and Diet in Health and Diseases, ..."it has been observed that coffee raises the blood pressure slightly, affects the heart activity and stimulation. Higher blood sugar levels have been reported more from the caffeine users than from the non-users. It affects the capability of the body and mind to cope up with tension-provoking situations. Caffeine is the most powerful of a group of stimulating alkaloid drugs known as Xanthines". It acts as a powerful diuretic (i.e. stimulates urination) and can interfere with sleep. A recent Dutch study shows that gallstone sufferers may experience abdominal pain after drinking coffee as black coffee sets off a squeezing movement in the gall-bladder by increased level of a hormone which causes this squeez in the gall-bladder.

4. Alcohol

Tension is nothing but an indicator of the aroused state of

affairs of a person. Alcohol is considered to be a drink which can be called stimulator and has direct bearing on creating an arousal state.

Alcohol has direct bearing on the nervous system which results in shutting off of rational mind during its peak arousal and hence this leads the consumer of alcohol to feel to be away from the realities and facts of life. Consumption of excessive alcohol cannot be considered to be the solution of a problem. Excessive consumption of alcohol in the long run has bad effect on health and may result in reducing the capacity of a person to bear stressful situations. High consumption of alcohol promotes "free radicals" in the body which are floating oxygen molecules which attack body cells sometimes triggering off cancer.

Several epidemiological and clinical studies have demonstrated that the daily alcohol consumption (more than 50 to 60 grams of ethanol) has vasopressor effect that increases blood pressure. Abstaining from alcohol normalises blood pressure.

The common illusion about alcohol is that it keeps an individual warm on a cold night but in reality alcohol by dilating blood vessels produces a false sense of warmth. Actually it impairs regulatory mechanisms and makes its consumer more prone to catching cold. Another misconception about alcohol is that it sharpens appetite. Alcohol in fact reduces appetite and the desire for essential food stuffs and leads to malnutrition. Another myth about alcohol is that it increases sexual pleasure and performance. Whereas the fact is that alcohol decreases inhibition and increases desire. It leads to less secretion of sexual hormone which upsets delicate balance of hormones and brain chemicals which leads to decreased sexual pleasure and performance.

The stomach wall absorbs alcohol almost immediately and sends it into the blood stream through which it is carried to the liver, heart, lungs and brain. It can cause inflammation of the stomach wall, gastritis, obesity and loss of appetite leading to imbalanced diet and vitamins deficiency. It impairs the efficiency of central nervous system, slows down thinking, making concentration difficult and impairs the ability to react quickly. It also leads to cirrhosis. Excessive alcohol consumption decreases the body's immune mechanism. The excessive consumption of alcohol and other cortical depressants temporarily controls tension but during withdrawal stage the autonomic nervous system becomes hyperactive. Against above, the findings of researchers on post-menopausal women, reported in the Journal of Alcoholism, reiterate that moderate consumer of alcohol showed higher level of estrogen levels than other women of their age. Estrogen helps in prevention of bone loss and heart disease.

5. Cigarette and Tobacco

It has been observed that when one is in an arousal position one starts smoking cigarettes excessively. Scientific studies have revealed that excessive consumption of cigarettes during stress is more on account of psychological reasons. Excess consumption of cigarettes may have a bad effect on health which reduces one's capability to deal effectively with stressful situations. Keeping in view the bad effects of cigarettes on health, a cigarette has also been defined as a roll of tobacco which has a flame at one end and a fool on the other. It can be said : life is yours, it is for you to live it or smoke it.

The human lungs need clean fresh air in order to oxygenate the blood. Polluting that air with tar and nicotine of tobacco smoke starves the blood of life giving oxygen. Smoke particles remain in the lungs forever gradually filling the tiny air tubes and clogging them thereby reducing the total capacity of the lungs. Cigarette smoking accelerates the formation of blockages in the heart's arteries. It is a major factor in erectile dysfunction and thereby affect sexual life. In terms of findings of the researchers of Emory School of Medicine, Atlanta, USA, damaged bones of smokers may take as much as five months longer to heal because nicotine and carbon monoxide hinder oxygen delivery and blood vessel development essential for repair.

The effects of smoking can be summarised as follows :

(a) It increases adrenaline flow.

(b) It speeds up heart beating rate.

(c) It constricts blood vessels.

(d) It makes blood more likely to clot.

(e) It increases the blood levels of fat and cholestrol.

(f) Tobacco smoke irritates the lining of stomach and makes it vulnerable to any attack by acid.

As per British Medical Journal, research studies show that nicotine addicts are more likely to develop premature cataract. John Hopkins University researchers have concluded that if one quits smoking, chances of prematurely developing cataract may be cut by as much as 50 per cent. Research studies by American Academy of Actuaries indicate that men who never smoke live longer than life long smokers by an average of 16 years. Research shows that many persons' minds and lives are messed up with fatal illusions that smoking makes one powerful, beautiful, attractive or sexy, ignoring that it may cause cancer, heart disease and other fatal diseases.

6. Drug Addiction

"When you take an addictive drug you are signing your death warrant".

With an easy availability of drugs in the market and indiscriminate prescription of drugs in general has led people to believe that a small capsule containing a drug is a panacea which contains in itself solution to all problems. In general one stretches one's hand to swallow a small pill to get rid of symptoms that a disease produces in a body as a warning signal. Naturopathy experts believe that drug is a tax on vitality. Drug removes symptoms of disease and creates an illusion of temporary relief.

The various bad effects of indiscriminatory use of drugs can be broadly classified as follows :

1. Drugs adversely affect vitamin metabolism.

2. They cause several biochemical and electrophysical changes in the brain tissue, that result in memory impairment, failing mental powers leading to confusion and severe disorientation.

3. There is no drug or chemical that is entirely free from the risk of causing liver damage. Barbiturates

may cause hepatitis (inflammation of the liver) and Cholestross (stoppage or suppression of the flow of bile).

4. Skin diseases
5. Cardiovascular diseases
6. Can folate deficiency
7. Withdrawal symptoms

Induced sleep by use of sleeping pill can give temporary relief but continuous use over a long period of time creates adverse psychological side effects. The latest research studies of the "The Citizen Health Research Group of USA" have confirmed the viewpoint and have concluded that the most widely prescribed pill in the U.S. market (i.e. Halcion) may be causing more anxiety, restlessness, amnesia, aggression and paranoia to its regular users over a long period of time.

7. Noise

Scientific studies have indicated that noise level in atmosphere directly affects one's capability in dealing with stressful situations. Exposure to noise over 90 decibels (measurement of intensity of sound) continuously for 10 minutes can produce damaging effects on hearing system. Sound louder than 100 decibels can even produce permanent damage to the hearing system. According to international Standard 65 db (decibles) is considered tolerable. Sounds arrive at inner hair, called cochlea. This spiral passage is lined with tens of thousands of cells with micro scopic hair on them. These are called cilia which vibrate in response to the sounds and transform the vibrations into electric signals that are pulsed to the area of the brain responsible for hearing. When loud noises bombard the ear, cilia flatten out and may take hours before they straighten out again. Repeated bombardment makes cilia die and a little bit of hearing also dies.

The Federal Health Agency of Germany has recently issued a report stating "The risk of a heart attack as a result of long-term exposure to traffic noise is substantially higher than that of contracting cancer as a result of exposure to asbestos dust. Two percent of heart attack cases are a direct result of traffic noise. "Constant exposure to loud noise can cause – dizziness, lack of concentration and possibility of mental imbalance. Noise can aggravate problem of the aged and the sick, hypertension, heart disease and vertigo. Symptoms that appear in the persons who are living in noise polluted area are as follows :

(a) Insomnia

(b) Fatigue

(c) Hypertension

(d) High blood pressure

(e) Deafness

(f) Diseases of circulatory disorders, nervousness.

Experiments have shown that increase in the noise levels has an inhibiting effect on alpha activity. Studies conducted in U.S.A. and Japan on school children show that children from noisy areas work more slowly, tire more quickly and also take longer to master tasks that require thought because of the damage done by noise to their power of concentration. In short it can be said that noise affects the ear's hair cells which are called stereocilia lined up inside a small, snail-shaped organ called the chochlea. These hair cells have very important role to play as these participate in the process stage of the complicated mechanism of hearing. In tension, less oxygen goes to these hair cells, if such tension continues for a long period of time, hearing gets affected.

8. Wrinkles

In tension, body goes into a survival mode, the blood supply that nourishes the skin diverts to vital organs, less supply of blood goes to the skin over a long period of time which leads to development of wrinkles. Tension lowers sex hormone production which produces natural skin oil. This has an important role to play to keep natural plasticity. This compels elastic fibres to break down and increases wrinkles.

Though tension is one of the factors which damages skin, other factors which damage skin include the exposure to ultraviolet rays of sun, diet, oxygen and blood circulation.

9. Behaviour Masking

"The World has enough of slaves of impurity but perhaps more dangerous are the slaves of purity concealing their weakness under the name of morality"

Thus said, **Swami Ram Tirath,** a great saint and seer of modern India.

Through the child rearing practices, social norms are taught to an individual. The enriched Indian culture which is known for its family ties, teaches children from the inception to mask their behaviour in the name of cultural practices, moral values and character which lead them to supress their emotions. The practice of not allowing the younger ones to argue with elders on rational ground leads to high level of tension which normally bursts out in the form of emotional imbalance or in destructive behaviour.

10. Menopause

Menopause is only a milestone in a woman's path and it normally occurs between the ages of 45 and 55 years. In this stage fewer follicles are stimulated and less amount of estrogen is released during each menstrual cycle.

For this reason the lining of the uterus is less satisfactorily stimulated and menstrual flow becomes less regular and less predictable. The quantity of blood gets less and the interval between two menstrual periods is usually increased. The co-ordinated control of menstruation which has been so effective since adolescence gets out of gear, as the controlling gland unwinds into a quieter phase of life.

The reduction in secretion of estrogen affects the tissues which make up the female genital tract and breasts. It has been observed that it is difficult for women to adjust in the start of puberty and adolescence; similarly many women find reducing tides of such hormones difficult to adjust to. This leads them to depression, fatigue and insomnia. The peculiar irregularity of the period may subconsciously increase her tension with the realisation that her physical and sexual attraction is waning. The feeling of old age is induced. This results in change in emotional balance leading to tension. It must be understood that it is a temporary phase which every woman undergoes. This change in life should not be taken as the end of the life, as such. A healthy outlook may check tension arousal.

11. Hair Growth

Hair health is a reflection of one's health. Tension contributes a lot to early grey hair and baldness, though the other factors on which the colour, length and texture of hair depends include hereditary factors and the diet that one takes.

The role of hair is to protect. It is immaterial whether the hair are at brows, eyelashes or the pubic place. Facial hair give warmth as compared to pubic and armpit hair which lessen chaffing in winter. Hair on scalp protect the head from sun's heat, infra-red rays and other rays in the atmosphere.

The part of hair which lies below the epidermis is called corium. Sebacious glands are attached to the follicle which are scattered throughout the body and these glands provide lubrication and keep the follicles moist. During tension the working of hormones and glands gets affected. When this working gets upset, the follicles stop moist producing material. This leads to fall of hair and the colour of hair also gets affected making it grey. Greying of hair and baldness often contribute to tension which can be controlled if the person maintains cool and poise.

6

MANAGEMENT STRATEGIES AND THERAPIES

Tension is one's physical, mental and chemical response to things that are frightening, confusing or irritating. In managing tension a person is confronted with two problems:

(a) To meet the requirements of tension.

(b) To protect the self from psychological damage and disorganization.

When a person feels competent to handle a tension provoking situation, his behaviour tends to be task oriented i.e. dealing with the requirements of adjustive demands. But when feeling of adequacy is seriously threatened by the tension, his reactions tend to be defence oriented i.e. protecting the self from hurt.

Coping has been defined broadly as any effort towards tension management or the things that people do to avoid being harassed by strain of life. One's cognitive and behavioural efforts constantly keep on changing so as to manage specific external or internal demands. The word manage includes minimizing, avoiding, tolerating and accepting the tension.

Any tension provoking situation can be faced by either task oriented reaction patterns or defence oriented reaction patterns. Task-oriented reaction patterns are aimed at meeting the demands of the tension provoking situations whereas defence oriented reaction patterns may involve making changes in one's self or one's surroundings or both depending on the situation only. Task-oriented reactions are based on objective appraisal of the situation. They are rational, constructive and consciously directed. Inaccurate information, faulty value and poor judgement can lead to mal-adaptive reaction.

Listed below are Ego-defence mechanisms which function to relieve tension and to protect the self from hurt and devaluation. These reactions protect individuals from internal and external threats.

(a) **Denial of reality :** Protection of self from unpleasant reality by refusal to perceive or face it.

(b) **Fantasy :** Gratifying frustrated desires by imaginary achievements.

(c) **Repression :** Preventing painful or dangerous thoughts from entering consciousness.

(d) **Rationalization :** Attempting to prove that one's behaviour is "rational" and justifiable and thus worthy of self and social approval.

(e) **Projection :** Placing blame for difficulties upon others or attributing one's own unethical desires to others.

(f) **Reaction formation :** Preventing dangerous desires from being expressed by exaggerating opposed attitudes and similar type of behaviour, using them as "barriers".

(g) **Displacement :** Discharging pent-up feelings usually of hostility, on objects less dangerous than those which initially aroused the emotions.

(h) **Emotional insulation :** Reducing ego involvement and withdrawing into passivity to protect self from hurt.

(i) **Intellectualization (isolation) :** Cutting off affective charge from hurtful situations or separating incompatible attitudes by logic-tight compartments.

(j) **Undoing :** Counteracting immoral desires or acts.

(k) **Regression** : Retreating to earlier developmental level involving less mature responses and usually of a lower level of aspiration.

(l) **Introjection** : Incorporating external values and standards into ego structure so that individual is not at the mercy of external threats.

(m) **Compensation** : Covering up weakness by emphasizing desirable trait or making up for frustration in one area by overgratification in another.

(n) **Acting out** : Reducing the anxiety aroused by forbidden or dangerous desires by permitting their expression. Tension produces multidimensional complexities and its solution lies no more within the domain of pychological techniques only. Rather, there is need to look into the mence of tension by philosophical approach, physical approach and medical curative approach also.

Time management concept tells us to have a time and place for everything and do everything in its time and place. This technique helps in getting optimum results and one finds more time for leisure as compared to those who are always hurrying. When one races with time and that too all the time, the racer ends up in the constant state of tension. It has been rightly said that being rushed is not a virtue but it is sign of bad management. Life would be simple indeed if one's biological and psychological needs were automatically gratified, but instead these turn out to be environmental and personal obstacles which place adjustive demands (stress) on the individual. Hence the demand is for proper planning and systematic and steady execution.

Proper time management helps not only in avoiding tension but also in developing an orderly mind that functions effectively and efficiently without confusion. Discipline has a vital role to play in reducing tension in day to day life. Discipline is orderly doing of things and by this process, the doer gets a lot of satisfaction in the long run. Jawaharlal Nehru, India's first Prime Minister has rightly emphasised that the greatest of all indisciplines is emotional indiscipline which upsets an individual the most. There is a growing conviction that the way people manage tension affect their psychological, physical and social well-being.

One can, by adopting correct managing strategy and therapy regarding the problem of tension, enjoy good health which is nothing but an orderly, unified and progressive functioning of the individual's physiology and psychology.

I. PHILOSOPHICAL APPROACH OF TENSION MANAGEMENT

RELIGION

Religion is the source of philosophy. It is concerned with the transformation of man's mind. It aims to intergrate the inner being of man – both his character, aspiration and his urges. The role of religion has been emphasised right from the origin of human being. Man has spent considerable amount of time, energy and money in exploring the outer world. The search has left him tense, stressful and at war with himself, his fellowmen and surroundings. This has led to the need to look inward to understand divine colours of universal brotherhood, love, peaceful dealings and harmonious interaction among ourselves under the supreme spiritual Fatherhood of single Soul. Religion has helped the mankind in exploring the miraculous powers that the right hemisphere of mind bears. This has been ignored in our formal education but nevertheless it has helped us to learn the technique of wisdom by emphasising spatial, intuitive, deductive, sympathetic and holistic approaches.

Religion helps an individual to restore, cohere and unite one's splintered being by making one realise the real self. It helps one to maintain equilibrium of mind so as to rise above desires. Religion has introduced the concept of real happiness by emphasising that sensual indulgence should not be taken as happiness. The causes of tension make one surrender and create a vaccum of happiness. When one realises the powers of innerself, the sources of tension are recognised in the form of one's greed, fear, jealousy, anger etc. Religion has emphasised the need to go for brain stilling as compared to brain storming by silencing powers. It has emphasized to go for interiorization by cleaning inner self rather than going for restorative activities in the form of drinking parties, aimless socializing and the like.

It has laid emphasis on surrender of lower ego to higher ego by realizing the stage of Sat-Chit-Anand : the state of All being, All knowledge, All bliss. It has imbibed in people the spirit of sacrifice for others. By the introduction of spirit of sacrifice and surrender of ego one can go above one's desires rather than falling in the web of desires which is the root cause of all tensions.

Religion develops the concept of faith which has been considered to be the strongest link in the path of learning. The pillar of all religions is faith. It is the faith in oneself, due to which others repose faith in us. When faith in one's own self develops it goes a long way in determining not only one's actions and behaviour, but also helps in stopping all sources of tension by generation of optimistic thinking. Let us pray in the words of Rabindra Nath Tagore :

"This is my prayer to Thee, my Lord,
Strike, strike at the roots of penury in my heart,
Give me the strength lightly to bear my joys and sorrows,
Give me the strength to make my love fruitful in service,
Give me the strength never to disown the poor or bend my knees before insolent might,
Give me the strength to raise my mind high above daily trifles,
Give me the strength to surrender my strength to Thee with love."

The ten tenets of religion, as enunciated by Manu, are Perseverance, equanimity, endurance, not to be lured, internal and external purity, control over senses, intellectual development, learning, truth in thought, word and deed, and abandoning of anger, which need to be propounded and practised.

The philosophical approaches in Hinduism are represented through the sacred books of

   (i) Mahabharata and the GITA in particular,

  (ii) Ramayana, and

 (iii) Vedas and allied scriptures

GITA AND TENSION

Mahatma Gandhi considered Gita as a potent source of tension control and mental poise. His words are clear and concise :

"When doubts haunt me, when disappointments stare me in the face and I see not one ray of hope on the horizon, I turn to Bhagavad Gita, and find a verse to comfort me, and immediately begin to smile in the midst of overwhelming sorrow".

The GITA, an epoch-making part of Mahabharata, has teachings which help in understanding the concept of happiness. It offers hope to mankind in all climes and a remedy in all situations. It is a guide for self-fulfilment, self-awareness, self evaluation for betterment. It is a practical manual that offers comprehensive advice to achieve 'moksha' by making one to understand the philosophy of this worldly life.

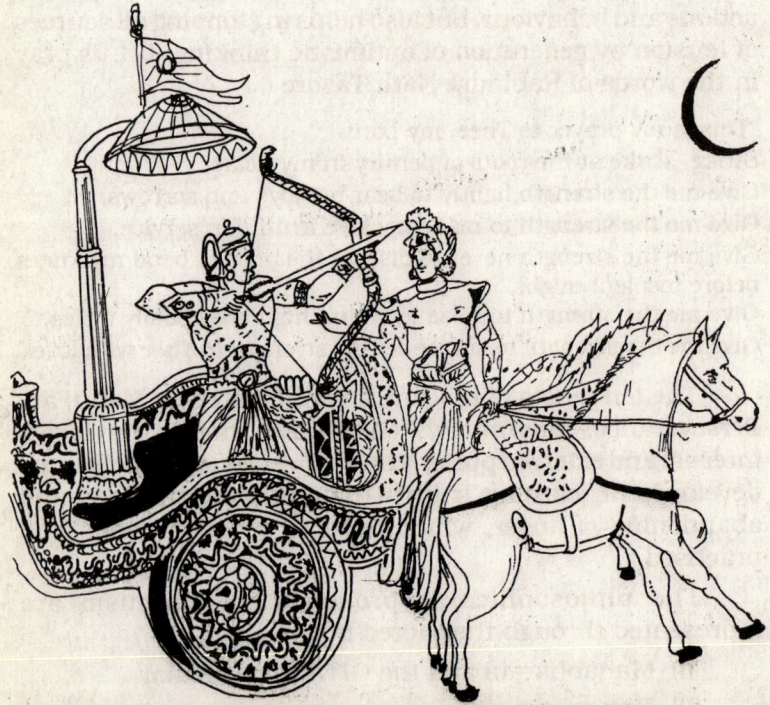

Fig. 6.1 : Lord Krishna revealing the essence of Gita as a tension management tool.

The teachings of Gita are the basic principles of life and if the same are pondered over in the right way, become a source of guidance to meet the various challenges of life.

1. It is necessary to surrender the lower unriped ego to higher riped ego through an intense inner self.

2. Uplift oneself through ownself, never bring it down.

3. Man is the creature of his faith, what his faith is that verifies what he is.

4. Work is important for purification of mind and intellectual work is important for cleaning of mind. This process of refinement has been called Chitta Shuddhi in GITA. In practice, purification through work means overcoming envy, greed, selfishness and similar tendencies of mind which may lead to tension. Actions may not bring happiness but there can't be happiness without actions. Inaction is like stagnant pond and work or action is like running water.

5. The flow of thought is governed by the messages one gets through five senses and this is manifested in the form of behaviour through speech and action. There is need to master one's desires born out of senses. Most of the problems are caused by desire, greed or craving. We give undue importance to the gratification of sensual and material desires. A man whose mind is free from desires of the senses under the discipline of the soul achieves external bliss.

6. Love every soul as Brahm dwells in every soul. Creator of this world and the source of happiness is within you. There is need of recognising Him which is possible when you are able to see him within you beyond the layers of artificiality. There is need to recognise the urge of developing unity of all living beings on spiritual platform.

"The supreme happiness comes to yogi when mind is peaceful, whose passions are at rest, who is sinless and is identified with God".   (*Sloka* 6.27)

Man's condition has been described like musk deer who does not know that musk is lodged right in the navel but it leaps and runs amuck all over the forest in search of the same.

7. When any work is done as duty and when the result is left to Him without attaching oneself with the result then only one can attain happiness. This emphasis needs full surrender before Him by developing full faith in Him.

"He who looks upon all as himself in pleasure or in pain is considered, O Arjun, a perfect yogi".

"He who does any work (service to humanity) and recognises me as the Supreme, who worships me without other attachments and who does not have hatred towards any creature, he reaches me, O Arjun."

One should not take credit for the success or failure, doer alone should not take the whole brunt himself (provided he has been doing consciously) and as such should not dissipate his energy in despair. Each individual can become a stitha-pragya through practice of rules.

The teachings of GITA cover very widely the problems of life and death, duty and devotion, action and inaction, knowledge and meditation and also provide eternal solution to the problems of mankind.

As per the teachings of GITA, Sat-Chit-Anand state is nothing but pure existence, consciousness and bliss. The root cause of all sufferings is on account of ignorance (avidya) and non-apprehension of reality (maya). Stitha-Pragya is a tension free person who is a personification of godliness.

RAMAYANA AND TENSION

Lord Rama set an example by leading a life of bare and pure minimum, even though he had access to the various facilities available to the prince of a kingdom. He emphasised on the art of enjoying life without becoming a slave of materialistic pleasures which are available in one's surroundings. It is the sole materialistic approach that has made people tiny creatures. There is need to rise above the body and the mind by driving oneself into the Divine powers. When one develops faith in Supreme Self, all tension disappears. There is need to conquer one's mind and become victorious. Rama advocated a life to be lived on pure heart, free from ego and pride.

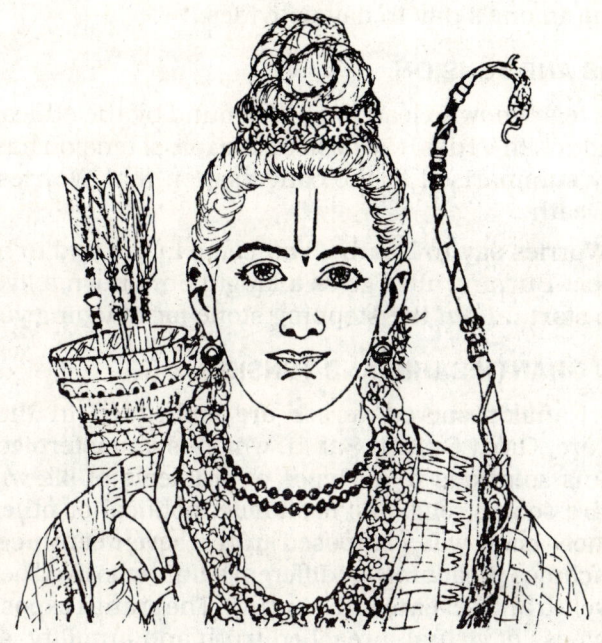

Fig. 6.2 : Lord Rama a model of tension-free individual.

The basic teachings of Ramayana, convey that one should lead the life of service, truth and love and these should not be touched by the sense of ego. It must be understood that Rama denotes ultimate knowledge. Hanuman is a medium through which Rama sent the message to the world. Shri Hanuman's life, the attitude of service, truth and love, all remained untouched by a sense of ego.

God has given everyone both intellect and faith so that one can apply the intellect in worldly matters and rely on faith in spiritual matters. In modern days this order has been reversed. People have started applying intellect in spiritual matters and rely on faith in worldly matters. Today one does every worldly thing on trust but when the question is about God, one often argues that until one can conceive God through intellect one can't beleive in God. Ramayana's teachings help us to overcome tension by introduction of the concept of faith, attitude of service, truth and rising above egoism, in one's day to day activities.

VEDAS AND TENSION

Vedas teach how to lead pure life bound by the ethical code of conduct. In Vedas, the destructive role of tension has been rightly summarised in the conversation that Worries have with Death :

Worries say to Death, "You come in the end to burn a corpse... Burning alive gives a laugh! So, I burn a live man in the start... I am the stepping stone for reaching you".

GURU GRANTH SAHIB AND TENSION

Guru Nanak's sacred verses are embedded in the holy scripture, Guru Granth Sahib, which is a masterpiece and contains solutions to all types of problems of life whether they are social, religious, economic, political or otherwise. This holy book was composed in the seventeenth century and includes preachings of different saints who lived between the twelfth and seventeenth century. The granth exposed the hollowness of virtual, preached truth and humility, spread the message of brotherhood. This covers very widely His voice against the social, religious and spiritual malpractices of the time and showed the path of happiness. Various teachings suggest the technique one should learn to overcome the tension provoking problems. One has to accept that it is basically one's attitude and outlook rather than an event that creates tension. The problem is universal as the words of Baba Sheikh Farid make evident:

"Farida main janea dukh mujh ku, dukh sabaia jag kothe char ke dekhia ghar ghar eh agg...."

(Guru Granth p. 1382)

(I thought as if I was the only unhappy man but when I looked around I found that every body is sailing in the same boat).

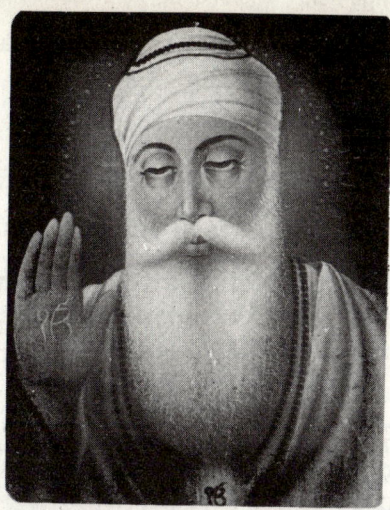

Fig. 6.3 : Guru Granth Sahib suggest ways and means to release tension.

The teachings of Guru Granth Sahib give a new dimension to solving various problems and warn aptly about the adverse effects of tension on body and mind which give birth to physiological, mental and neurological diseases.

"Jin ko chinta bahut bahut dehi veape rog...."

(Guru Granth p. 70)

(One who worries gets numerous diseases)

This sacred book while covering social problems, has rightly emphasised that a person does not become superior merely by caste, creed, colour, the family in which he takes birth or the riches. Superiority is not determined merely on the basis of religion that one adopts. A man is basically superior by actions. Casteism is one of the causes of tension and has been dealt in the following quotations :

(a) "Phakker jati phakkar naon...."

(Raga Malhar, Guru Nanak p. 83)

(Caste is a condemnable notion and so is pride of name)

(b) "Garbh ras main kul nahin jati ...."

(Raga Guari, Kabir p. 324)

(In the mother's womb one belongs neither to a dynasty nor to a caste)

The need to give respect to female class has been emphasised. For this Guru Nanak says,

"So kyun manda akhiya jitt
Janme rajan...."

(Guru Nanak p. 473)

(Why revile one who has given birth to kings)

Similarly, when all life has originated from one common source, the Supreme Power, how any one can be bad.

Regarding economic problems, Guru Nanak's teachings preach the need to

(a) Reduce one's needs to match with one's capacity.

(b) Be contended with what one has, when one hasn't had those things that one likes.

Humanity and service without selfish motive have been prescribed to overcome the evils of pride, anger, avarice, jealousy, revenge, hatred etc. Many of the problems that arise out of anger can be overcome by developing the quality of forgiveness and tolerance. The need to develop the quality of silence to overcome many of our problems has been emphasised.

To have good health, this sacred granth suggests less sleep, less eating and less clothing.

"Dhrig Dhrig khaea
Dhrig Dhrig soia
Dhrig Dhrig kapad ang charaja...."

(Guru Granth p. 796)

Guru Granth Sahib's teachings suggest the need to develop the technique of solving problems by way of compromise and adjustment.

"Ek ne kahi, dusre ne mani
Nanak kahe dono giani".

The need to develop the role of charity and having faith in God has also been emphasised in the teachings. His name alone works as a panacea to many problems. In Todi Mahala 5(713), it has been suggested to sing the virtues of the Lord to get peace, poise, fortitude and the secret knowledge thus obtained helps in eradicating all sorrows. Churn His name with steady mind to avoid loss of butter. Guru Nanak has advised to learn virtue of five elements viz. to learn patience from earth, coolness or calmness from the water, equanimity from the air, all embracing or pervasive qualities from the sky and purity from the fire. In terms of Maru Mohala 5 Ghara 4 Ashtapadian (1018),

> Supreme light is that light of the Lord that illumine the corridor of my heart.

> Supreme worship is the name worship of the Lord.

> Supreme renunciation is the surrender of body and mind unto Lord and also of lust, anger, greed, attachment, ego etc.

> Best begging is begging for singing of the virtues of God through Guru's teachings.

> Best awakening is possible by singing the glories of Lord.

> Best clinging is clinging the holy feet of Guru i.e. adopting the qualities of Almighty.

> Best refuge is the refuge of Lord.

It is only when the Supreme infinite, omnipotent, omnipresent, omniscient, immaculate Lord showers His mercy on an individual only, he is released from all the bonds. He alone can take one across the ocean of the world of conflict, pain, greed and attachment.

BUDDHISM AND TENSION

Just as the sea is never satiated even with thousands of rivers and fire with fuel frequently added to it, so is an individual not satisfied with all sensual pleasures. In terms of teachings of Buddhism, there is need for complete destruction of three drives which give birth to human tension. They are cravings for :

(a) pleasure

(b) existence

(c) prosperity

A man becomes free, when he goes for right belief and aspiration, right speech and conduct, right livelihood and endeavour, right memory and meditation. The fact is that birth, decay, illness, death, separation are nothing but sufferings which lead to tension.

He has attained peace who is indifferent to the pleasures of the senses, who has traversed the mire without getting besmirched. He has no son, no relatives, no land, no wealth. Their ownership does not please him; he is free of jealousy, of greed, this saintly man abjures pride, he does not think mean, he does not compete. The web of time does not bind him. He too does not weave a web for anyone. He is indifferent, does not lament a loss, does not worry. Such a one has attained Nirvana.

Buddha : Suttanipat

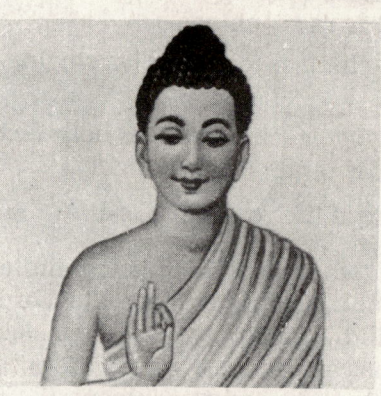

Fig. 6.4 : Lord Buddha "Desires are the main cause of tension".

When one is not able to obtain what he desires, he is led to tension. Desires give birth to fear and grief. The need to abandon all desires has been emphasised in the teachings of Lord Buddha by adopting seven methods.

(a) **By insight :** This is done by overcoming the delusion of self, right along hesitation and dependence on external rites.

(b) **By subrogation :** of the five senses and mind.

(c) **By right use :** of clothes, alms and abode.

(d) **By endurance :** in all situations whether they are painful or pleasurable.

(e) **By avoiding :** dangers, improper places and bad companions.

(f) **By removal :** of evil thoughts.

(g) **By cultivation :** of higher wisdom.

Actions, physical, verbal or mental, must be controlled and the direction for the same is considered correct if it leads to happiness. There is need to do meritorious acts from all the faculties called faith, energy, awareness, concentration and knowledge. Buddhist path suggests the path of truth consisting of morality, concentration and wisdom. The path is considered good if it avoids self-mortifying austerities and self deceiving in sensual pleasures. The path suggested by Lord Buddha believes in the doctrine of friendlines and charity, of renunciation and concentration, of wisdom and compassion, of morality and purity. The noble path consists of eight constituents viz. right view, right aspiration, right speech, right action, right livelihood, right effort, right mindfulness and right concentration. His teachings are aimed to create universal love without giving any weight to divisive forces of caste or creed. For getting true happiness, he suggested to observe the following rules of morality :

(a) Abstinence from taking life.

(b) Abstinence from theft.

(c) Abstinence from adultery.

(d) Abstinence from telling lies.

(e) Abstinence from taking intoxicating things.

(f) Abstinence from eating at the wrong hour.

(g) Abstinence from enjoying vulgar shows such as dancing, singing and instrument playing.

(h) Abstinence from using ornaments.

(i) Abstinence from sleeping on a high (luxurious) bed.

(j) Abstinence from borrowing.

(k) Abstinence from slander.

(l) Abstinence from impolite speech.

(m) Abstinence from talking senselessly.

(n) Abstinence from covetousness (greediness).

(o) Abstinence from malevolence (ill will).

(p) Abstinence from false views.

It is craving for self enjoyment in this life and even thereafter, one leads a life of tribulation, grief, suffering, distress and despair between life and death and only by following the path suggested one can have the real bliss.

BIBLE AND TENSION

Bible has emphasised the need to develop faith in Him and this therapy does wonders to get rid of all diseases including tension. Bible is considered to be a philosophy, a system of theology, of metaphysics and of worship. It contains moral and ethical code, techniques and formulae to understand human nature. By development of faith in Him, by infusing positive thoughts of hope, faith, courage, expectancy and by getting rid of old, dead thoughts of fear, one can tap wonderful effects that stem from one's mind.

The secret behind tension is that human mind is literally saturated with apprehensive thoughts, defeat thoughts, gloomy thoughts etc. which ultimately become a part of the sub-conscious mind and repeatedly the sub-conscious ideas reach the conscious zone and make the individual tense again and again. If one's mind is saturated with the ideas of faith, hope, happiness and glory, one automatically attains a tension-free life. One needs to drain out thoughts of fear and failure which lead to tension and replace the same with new dynamic faith in Him. Such faith gives peace, cleans the mind and develops determination. Spiritual faith in Him conserves the energy for clarity of thoughts and appropriate actions.

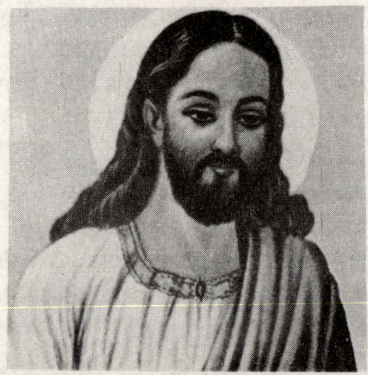

Fig. 6.5 : Jesus Criste "Unquestionable faith in Him leads to tension free life.

The following preachings of the Bible, emphasise the need to develop unquestionable faith in Him, to attain tension-free life.

1. "If ye have faith .... nothing shall be impossible upto you". (*Mathew* 17 : 20)

2. "I can do all things through Christ, which strengthen them". (*Philipiam* 4 : 13)

3. "Ye shall know the truth and the truth shall make you free. Get the truth into your mind and you will be free of such failures." (*John* 8:32)

4. "If you have faith as a grain of mustard seed .... nothing shall be impossible upto you".

   (*Mathew* 17:20)

5. "Submit yourselves therefore to God. Resist the devil and He will free you". (*James* 4.7)

6. "....don't be anxious about tomorrow for tomorrow will be anxious for itself. Let the days own trouble be sufficient for the day" (*Mt.* 634)

7. Jesus says that the human beings who are weary should come to Him and lay all the burden on Him..... He will bear it. In his famous sermon on the mount. He calls the individual to be merciful, peace loving, righteous and pure at heart.

QURAN AND TENSION

The holy Quran advocates purification of soul and reconstructing society based on this. It denounces concept of religion, Muslims are those who keep up prayer (Salah), pay the welfare due (ZAKAT), command what is proper and forbid what is improper. In Islam all men are equal irrespective of their colour, language, race or nationality. Teachings address to the conscience of mankind. Islam aims at establishing equilibrium between the two aspects of life viz. the material and the spiritual. It says that everything in this world is for man but man is himself for the service of higher purpose the establishment of moral and just order which fulfills the will of GOD. Its teachings cater for the spiritual as well as the temporal needs of men.

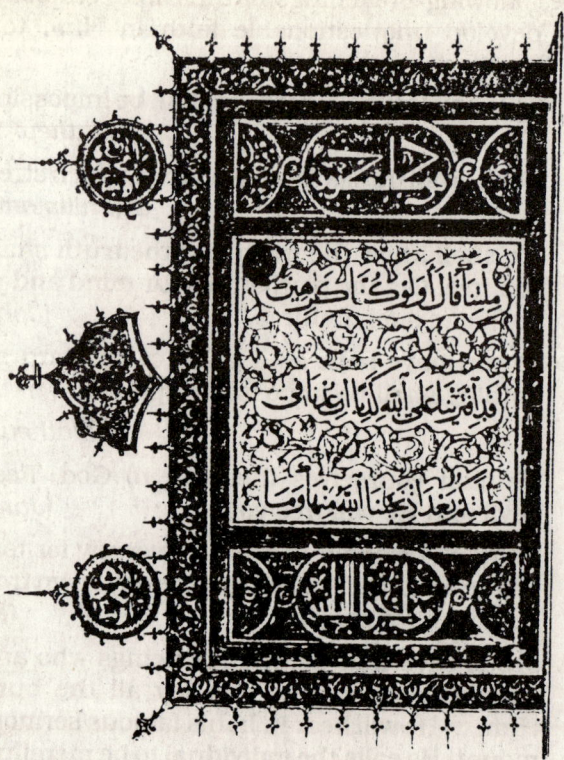

Fig. 6.6 : Muslims believe that the Koran is the last and most perfect of God's revelations to humankind. The Koran is made up of 114 Surahs, or chapters each of which consists of one or more verses, known as ayahs.

The code of life, has been envisaged in the two documents called 'Shar'ah' in Islamic terminology :

(a) The holy book in which God has expounded His law viz. Quran and

(b) The authoritative interpretation and exemplification of the book of God as given by various prophets through their words and deeds by setting practical example in their capacity as the messenger of God and last on Mohammad (peace be upon him).

As per this if one follows the teachings of Islam, he is likely to get peace, will be away from tension. According to Islamic law man is trustee, "Khalifah" of God. All are the

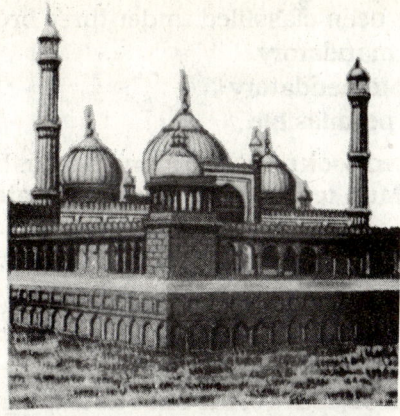

Fig.6.6 : Mosque a place which helps in tension reduction.

creations of God and a man is expected to voluntarily acknowledge this fact by maintaining loyalty and allegiance to Lord. Man should renounce his claim of supremacy to Allah. Man or his actions and thoughts should gracefully accept that all powers and organs, rather all free will functions are gifts from Him. Independence of choice itself has been accrued to man by Him and all the things in which man's will operates belong to him. All those persons who surrender themselves to the will of God and community so formed is called Muslim Society. It is God and not man whose will is the primary source of law in the Muslim society.

Man has not been left like a ship without moorings who is supposed to be tossed about by the blow of wind and tides. As HE is all wise, all powerful and Omniscient man is expected to follow His guidance to achieve his bliss. The holy Quran and prophet's guidance cover practically all fields of life right from cradle-to grave. A person following the guidance as provided by Him is to get Divine pleasure He gets eternal peace as he follows His will against the actions motivated by personal motives of worldly man. A man is expected to adopt an attitude which is approved by God. In Islam spiritual development is nearness to God. The main features of Islam can be summed up as follows :

1. The sacred book reveals to man how to live life by nurturing the good. This has been termed as Marufat and has been classified under three broad categories.
   (a) The mandatory
   (b) Recommendatory
   (c) The permissible

   The sacred book reveals to man what has been prohibited i.e. the Munkarat, under two broad categories.
   (a) Absolutely prohibited i.e. HARAM
   (b) Those things which have been disliked and discourage

   The shar'ah is a complete plan of life embracing in it social order.

2. The main objective of the Shar'ah is to construct human life on the basis of marufat (virtues) and to cleanse it of the munkarat (vices).

3. Besides setting standards. Islam furnishes man with the means of determining good and evil conduct.

4. The moral code of Islam covers smallest details of domestic life as well as broad aspects of national and international behaviour. It integrates through its teachings moral virtues by prescribing their limits and utility, and assigning to them their proper place.

5. The three sanctions on the back of moral law as envisaged in Islam are as follows :
   (a) the love and fear of God
   (b) the sense of accountability on the day of judgement
   (c) the promise of external bliss and reward in life.

6. The meaning of worship must be extended to beyond mere rituals into all activities as it regulate all aspects of life. Two important aspects of worship are :
   (a) There should be feeling of absolute certainty and conviction in ones heart about the God i.e. Allah.
   (b) A man should seek His guidance in every stir of one's conscience, in every fluttering of the senses and in every movement of life.

7. To do one's duty it is not bad to remember one's right alongwith duties and also not forgetting the right of others.

8. It is not possible to oppress women, children, old people, sick persons or the wounded. Woman's honour and ch. sity are worthy of respect in all circumstances.

9. According to Islam the real spirit of marital life is love, understanding and mutual respect. The most fundamental institution of human society is the unit of family. For proper regulation of life, Islam has imposed regulations of Hijab (for muslim woman), ban on free mixing of men and women, restrictions on filthy music and pictures. Discouragement of the spread and propagation of obscenities and aberrations.

10. Islam gives importance to neighbours. He wishes man to share one's happiness and sorrows with neighbour, though overall one's friendship and enmity should be for the pleasure of God only. Cold shoulders to neighbour has been looked down by Quran. As per Him a person is not true muslim who takes his fill while his neighbour starves.

11. Equal opportunities to every one : Islam believes in equality in respect of the opportunities for the struggle for securing a livelihood and for claiming the uppermost rung of the ladder of well being and prosperity. The idea is to create love and affection among the people.

12. Items which create disharmony have been discouraged.
Islamic laws categorically hold as illegal, manufacture and sale of liquor and other intoxicants, adultery, professional dancing and obscenities, gambling, speculation, races and lotteries (transactions of speculative nature, price manipulation by withholding the sale of necessities of life.)

13. Islamic law permits only descent life but one can't waste one's riches on luxurious pursuits.

"Eat and drink but don't be extravagent" The Quran **

14. As per Islamic laws the real place for growth, upliftment and elevation of the spirit lies in the midstream of the activity of life and not in solitary places of spiritual hibernation. Body is not a prison house for soul but its workshop or factory. It stands not for life denial but for life fulfillment. It does not expect to avoid material

things but spiritual elevation is to be achieved by living piously in the rough and tumble of life and not by renouncing the world. The prophet said : A Muslim who lives in the midst of society and bears with patience the affliction that comes to him is better than the one who shuns society and can't bear any wrong done to him.

15. Road to spirituality : Three pillars of the road are as follows :

   (a) Islam (Faith) : To have unreserved faith through intellect and his will, holding high in the head and heart of a man for God taking Him as the only master, sovereign and deity.

   (b) Ita'at (Obedience) meaning that a man divests himself of his independence altogether and accepts subservience of God in practice after having proclaimed faith in him and his creed.

   (c) Taqwa (Piety) : It consists in a practical manifestation of the faith in God in the mode of daily life. It is desisting from everything which He does not approve.

16. The path of spiritual development is not meant for individuals only but for the communities and nations as well.

17. All human beings are equal and constitute one fraternity. They will not be subjected to any racial, national or class distinctions of any kind. No one will be regarded as high or low.

18. Knowledge : Quran gives lot of importance to gaining more knowledge :

   (a) "Those who have no knowledge are not equal to those have it (39:9 the Quran).

   (b) "Basic qualification for leadership among other things are knowledge and physical strength (2:247 The Quran).

   (c) It is by virtue of knowledge that man is superior to angles and has been made vicegerent of God on earth (2:30 the Quran)

   The Quran gives complete code of life not only for individual but for the society and if principles of life are properly understood and obeyed, one is likely to get eternal peace, The mechanism of spiritual training which Islam has laid for preparing individuals and society for this purpose are as :

1. **Faith :** Three basic articles of Islamic faith are :
   (a) Belief in Oneness of God
   (b) Belief in the prophethood of Muhammad (peace be upon him) and in the guidance which he bequeathed; and
   (c) Belief in life after Death and in man's accountability before God on day of Judgement.

   All these beliefs and concepts are epitomised in the Kalimah "There is no God but Allah; Muhammad is His Prophet"

   In this regard, the Qur'an says

   "Those who believe and act righteously, joy is for Him, and blissful home to return to"

   (13:29)

   And the Prophet Muhammad (peace be upon him) said;
   "God does not accept belief if it is not expressed in deeds, and does not accept deeds if they do not conform to belief".

   The test of acceptance of God and His Prophet lies in conducting all human affairs in accordance with the law revealed by them.

2. **Prayer (Salah) :** Which brings man into communion with God five times a day receiving His remembrance reiterating His fear, developing His love, reminding man of the Divine commands again and again. The prayer is offered in congregation which inculcates social discipline, awakens a sens of social responsibility in man, organises human rights in a society. The idea is that society as a whole prepares them for the spirtual development.

3. **Zakat (Jihad) :** Islam by making it obligatory for rich to share total accumulated wealth 2½ % pa, in agriculture land depending totally on natural for water and other on irrigation respectively commands 10% & 5% of agriculture produce toward ZAKAT. By this Islam develops the sense of monetary sacrifice, sympathy and co-operation among the people. The real meaning of Zakat is sublimity and purification.

4. **Fasting (Soum) :** This is observed for a full month every year which trains a man individually and the Muslim

community as a whole in piety and self restraint. It enables to have experience of the pangs of hunger to both rich and poor. It prepares the people to undergo hardships to seek the pleasure of God.

5. **Hajji (Pilgrimage)** : This aims at fostering universal brotherhood of the faithful as the basis of worship of God.

II. PSYCHOLOGICAL APPROACH TO TENSION MANAGEMENT

Adverse life situations of an individual with poor emotional outlet lead to diminished ability to effectively sublimate or dissipate an emotional situation and it is likely to result in tension. It is also possible that adverse life situations may directly precipitate high tension level, but these manifestations are more likely to be found in those who have poor emotional outlet. Intensity of tension is not only determined by a situation in which an individual is surrounded, i.e. the stressors, but also by an individual's personality make-up. Different approaches suggested by applied psychologists and parapsychologists that increase an individual's tension-bearing capacity have been sumarised here by covering yoga, meditation, hypnosis, cognitive therapy, bio-feedback, music, laughter, recreation, colour therapy, acting, silence etc.

YOGA AS A TENSION REDUCTION TECHNIQUE

Yoga brings higher and more accomplished state of mind which transcends man's usual and everyday experience and opens for him a new field of vision. According to Swami Sivanand, Yoga is a synthetic technique embodying not only the various methods which thoroughly rejuvenate the body, maintain its vigour, and vitality, regulate the outgoing tendencies of the mind. It augments the intellectual capacity and leads to meditation. The Asanas and the Pranayama purify the body of the practitioner and make him fit to undertake meditation. Meditation opens the avenues of intuitional knowledge, makes the whole psychological nature of man calm, steady, luminous by awakening an ecstatic feeling. This brings an individual in contact with the source of Supreme Purusha, a contact in which lies the ultimate fulfilment of human life to bring endless joy and perfection.

Yoga and drugs, both act as tools to heal the ferocious disease called tension but there lies a basic difference between the two methods :

(a) Drugs prevent the brain from receiving the stimulus from any organ of the body, whereas the Yoga increases endurance capacity by effecting the central nervous system.

(b) Most of the drugs create negative side-effects, whereas yoga creates no bad effects.

Patanjali, father of Yoga, has suggested the following steps which form part of yoga to liberate man from sorrow and to obtain desired physical and mental levels :

1. **Yama :** Control and discipline by self-restraint.
2. **Niyama :** Rules, methods and principles.
3. **Asanas :** Making body postures.
4. **Pranayam :** Kriya with air through breathing.
5. **Pratyahara :** Avoidance of undesirable action.
6. **Dharana :** Concentration.
7. **Dhyana :** Meditation.
8. **Samadhi :** Contemplation.

1. Asanas

Various body postures (asanas), which help an individual to augment tension bearing capacity, are :

(a) **Shavasana :** Shavasana is a process of relaxing the whole body including brain and various systems. Relaxation is induced throughout the body in this pose which has beneficial impact on blood circulation. In this no peripheral resistance is encountered. Peripheral resistance is one of the causes of hypertension, i.e. high blood pressure. Failure to attain relaxation may result in insomnia and various neurosis problems.

(b) **Yoga-nindra :** Yoga nindra can be considered as the next stage of shavasana because it is considered to be the entry into layers of consciousness. Yoga-nindra helps in calming down of mind, slowing down heart beat, leads to less consumption of oxygen, normalises blood pressure, alpha waves increase and thereby relaxation is achieved. Shavasana is considered adequate if the same is undertaken for five to fifteen minutes whereas yoga-nindra is required to be undertaken for minimum ten minutes and may be extended to an hour.

(c) **Surya namaskar :** It is a chain of systematic body postures which helps in reducing physical and mental tension. This asana increases cardiac activity and helps in better flow of blood throughout the body. It tones up the nervous system by successively stretching the spinal column. The functioning of para-sympathetic and sympathetic nervous system becomes more acute.

(d) **Paschimottan asana :** This asana helps in strengthening Susukshmna nadi which normalises the functioning of nervous system and increases mind's capacity.

(e) **Halasana :** This asana is useful in reducing tension as it is very effective in increasing mental and physical energy. Through the practice of this asana one can learn to obtain the stage of hypnotic trance where extra-sensory perception become possible which calms the mind and cuts the roots of tension.

(f) **Sarvangasana :** As the name suggests, all parts of the body get benefitted by this asana. Nervous system gets toned up which makes a person more capable of handling day to day problems.

2. Pranayama and Tension

Pranayama is more than a mere breathing exercise which is the collecting, storing and conscious control of the vital pranic energies in one's body. Prayanama is a specific day of inhaling and exhaling breath. The three day of controlling breath in pranayama are as follows :

1. Pooraka : Filling the breath.
2. Rechaka - Throwing the breath out.
3. Kumbaka - Rolding the breath in or out.

The art of pranayama is the ladder of mental peace. It restores calmness and equipoise of the disturbed mind and helps in enhancing self-confidence. By pranayama one can change breath quality and thereby positive emotions can be created in the body. Some of the pranayamas which help in reducing tension are :

1. Shawans-presha pranayama.
2. Chandra-bhedhi pranayama.

3. Bhramari-pranayama.
4. Nadi-shodhan pranayama.
5. Sheetli-pranayama.
6. Kapal-bhati pranayama.

3. Bandhas as Tension Reliever

When pranayama exercises are practised with breath retention of more than ten seconds, there arises a need to complement them with bandhas. Three types of bandhas help in optimum consumption of oxygen that an individual inhales. The advantage of different bandhas can be summarised as follows:

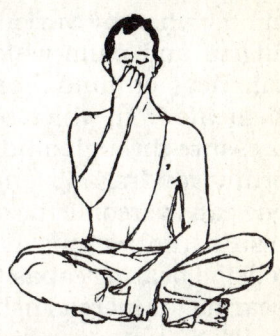

Fig. 6.8 : Sitting posture for the practice of Prana-yama.

(a) **Moola Bandha :** This is per-formed by contracting the rectum upward. This bandha helps in giving strength to inner muscles and activates their functioning. This bandha has a very beneficial effect on nervous system which increases the capacity of a person to bear and control tension producing factors.

(b) **Uddiyan Bandha :** This is done by exhaling the breath and by contracting the belly inwards. When exhaling is done all impure air from lungs is thrown out to make way for fresh air through inhaling. This bandha removes waste by increasing the blood flow near kidneys and near about parts.

(c) **Jallandhar Bandha :** This is performed by pressing the chin about three-four inches above the heart in the hollow form in the neck. This bandha helps in creating beneficial effect on the nervous system and the cortex, i.e. breathing control system. This affects 'Vasomotar' nerve and places pressure on heart.

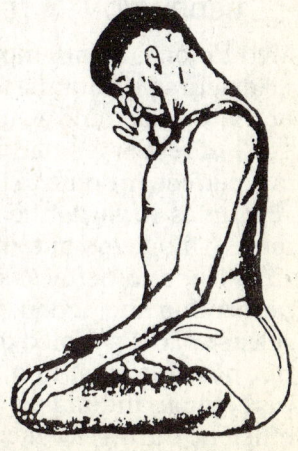

Fig. 6.9 : Jalandhar Bandh.

4. Mudras as Tension Reliever

Mudras represent combined poses of different fingers of hands whereby various levels of pressure are created on fingers and palm which have the effect of increasing the calmness of mind. Four fingers and thumb represent five elements from which body is said to be created. By creating pressure through mudras like vayu mudra, shunya mudra, prithvi mudra, aapaan mudra, prana mudra, lekhni mudra, one can overcome the deficiency of different elements which result into various diseases in body and thus increase tension bearing capacity. Various mudras which have direct bearing on increasing tension endurance are :

(a) **Gyan Mudra (first finger and thumb)** : In this mudra, pressure is created on the upper portion of palm, this result into subsiding the agitated feelings. This mudra has direct bearing on mental faculty. It removes uncertainty, insecurity anger, fear which create tension.

(b) **Shanti Mudra (Pressure on nose with second finger)** : This mudra as the name suggests help in bringing calmness of mind and subside agitated feeling created by anger.

Chapter 7 describes yoga as a tool of tension management in detail.

MEDITATION : A TENSION REDUCTION TECHNIQUE

Meditation is an attempt to still the mind through of stopping all discursive thinking to enable the higher level of conscious or the 'budha mind' to function. Meditation helps in bringing state of rest or a stage where there is least excitement. Rest is a perfect antidote to tension which allows to normalise its resources towards the resolution of any disorder that may arise. This helps in toning up the nervous system which in turn leads to better coordination between mind and body, perception and action. Deep rest during meditation helps in release of deep rooted tension and strain which otherwise is not possible even in a state of sleep. It helps in improving perception and makes the mind more creative, orderly and efficient during awakened state. Elimination of impurities becomes more effective during meditation. Deep state of rest created through meditation brings beneficial effects which can be summarised under three broad headings.

    (a) Physiological changes.

    (b) Biological changes.

    (c) Electro-physiological changes.

(a) **Physiological changes :** Physiological changes that come after meditation are such that they physiological rejuvenation by dissolving the effects of fatigue and tension. Research studies have established that meditation helps in reduction of oxygen consumption, carbon dioxide elimination, arterial lactae and its concentration, the decrease in heart rate, respiration rate brings rapid rise in skin resistance, abundance in alpha wave activity, and Symphony in contral and frontal derivation with occasional frontal theta wave. Studies have also established that blood flow indicates reduced sympathetic activity and reduced metabolic rate.

(b) **Biological changes :** The practice of meditation brings decline in plasma cortisol and lactae level, and significantly increases in the concentration of plasma phonlalanine and prelactin.

(c) **Electro-physiological changes :** During meditation it has been scientifically established that the spreading of large amplitude alpha waves take place in the interior region of brain.

Electro Myographic changes (EMG) : Frontal muscle activity is considered to be a physiological measure of anxiety. EMG shows that during and after the mediatation muscular activity and tension get reduced.

Meditation helps in creating state of deep relaxation which increases the ability of the individual to resist environmental stress. It increases physiological stability and adaptability of the nervous system which allows relaxation. It has been established that meditation produces beneficial effects in hypothalamus (a part of the brain) which is the centre that regulates and coordinates autonomic functions, secretes hormones, regulates appetite and temperament, and helps in controlling responses of Viscera. This is considered to be the major relay mechanism between cerebrum and autonomic centre. This, in turn effects the quality of sleep. The regulating mechanism in the hypothalamus has its own contribution in reducing or in increasing the tension level. Phycho-neurogenic factors operating through the cerebral cortex increase/decrease tension level. By controlling hypothalamus inner harmony can be brought. Endocrine glands, harmonal balance, autonomic nervous system, the viseral functions all are dependant on the working and production of hypothalamus. The fall in blood lactate during meditation brings in calmness and reduction in tension level. Meditation produces lasting effects in tension reduction as it goes deep into subconscious level by way of purification of mind.

Effects on Alpha, Beta, Delta waves During Meditation

Alpha is one of the electrical energies produced by the brain and can be measured by an electro-encephalograph (EEG). The rhythm of this energy is measured in cycles per second (CPS). Normal relaxed mind with eyes closed produces waves, with a frequency of 8 to 13 cycles per second. These waves disappear when one's eyes are opened. Generally about 14 CPS and up are called Beta waves, about 7 to 14 CPS are called Alpha waves, about 4 to 7 CPS are called Theta waves, below 4 waves are called Delta waves. Alpha waves usually appear in a relaxed mental state of a person, beta waves during intense mental activity, theta waves are more commonly seen in infants and delta waves during stupor, sleep or surgical anaesthesia. One can do different things in Alpha than one can do in Beta state. At lower frequencies brain receives and stores more information. The problem is to keep the mind alert at these frequencies which are associated more with day dreaming and sleep than with practical activity. The more one meditates the more it helps one to go deeper to control mind which increases body's healing power and restores the energy that one squanders on tension.

Meditation has been suggested by different experts in their own ways, but close inspection of all the different meditative techniques clearly indicats that virtually all types of meditation involve physical immobility and some form of perceptual concentration. The only difference observed in different techniques is target of concentration which can be an object, an idea, mantra or breathing.

There are several ways to do meditation. Some of the prominent techniques suggested by different experts are summarised here :

1. Rajneesh Meditation

Osho Rajneesh has given 112 methods of meditation which mainly differ in the constitution but all of them emphasise on:

- (i) Relaxation,
- (ii) Watchfulness and
- (iii) Non-judgemental attitude.

The first stage is a relaxed state in which the subject neither makes a conscious effort to control the mind nor stress on concentration. The second stage involves watching with a relaxed awareness what is going on without any interference. It is watching the mind silently without any judgement or evaluation. Then comes the stage when silence descends and movement ceases. In one of the commonly used technique out of the various techniques suggested by him for meditation, the following five steps are suggested :

The first step involves throwing out the garbage of mind by a let go approach and is done by jumping up and down vigorously, shouting, yelling and screaming, even obscenities if one likes, whatever comes in one's mind.

This is followed by shouting 'Hoo Hoo Hoo' until one gets totally exhausted. After this, one stands quietly and tries to experience the inner voice. Then in the 4th stage, long session of Sufi dancing takes place. Fifth and final stage allows one's creative energy to flow by observing silence.

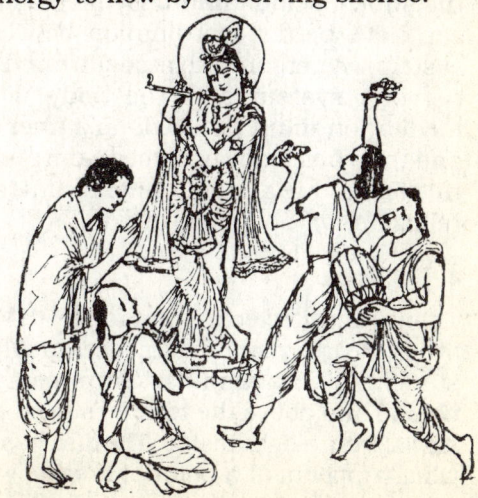

Fig. 6.10 : An ISKCON Group busy in Meditation.

2. ISKCON – The Society for Krishna Consciousness

This meditation technique suggests that chanting many times of the maha mantra "Hare Krishna" can lead one to realization of God and release of tension.

3. Transcendental Meditation

This type of meditation has been suggested by Maharshi Mahesh Yogi. It consists of repeating a given meaningless mantra which is supposed to possess a special sound quality which pacifies the mind. It stops the distracting thoughts and produces a state of relaxation in which the brain registers alpha waves, indicating a state of "Calm-awareness". It is a technique for experiencing a thought at the initial stages of development and enables the conscious mind to arrive systematically at the source of thoughts. It is a technique for expanding conscious awareness and for reducing tension. The word 'transcendental' means "going beyond". This technique takes the practitioner beyond the familiar level of wakeful experience to a state of profound rest coupled with heightened awareness. The process of thinking starts from the deepest level of consciousness and becomes grosser as it develops. Eventually it becomes gross enough to be perceived on the surface level of consciousness, the ordinary level of thinking. In this technique subconscious area of the mind is made conscious. This is done by consciously experiencing the thought in its infant state in the subconscious mind. By increasing conscious level one can have better coordination between mind and nervous systems. A person with anxious mind, exhausts and irritates nervous system and the body. During transcendental meditation mind proceeds to a finer state wherein thought and the whole body becomes calm and quiet. After mastering this technique a practitioner levitates or flies which leads to relaxation of body and mind.

4. Raj Yoga

This meditation technique is of BRAHMA KUMARIS. It consists of high degree visual experiences taught in small groups where students sit in a semi-darkened room facing the teacher. Just behind and above the teacher's head is a red plastic disc that glows, from a light inside. The disc has a tiny hole in the centre which appears at a point of intense white light, representing the Supreme Soul – Shiv Baba. The student thinks of himself as a bodiless (Asharir) and visualizes the light and power is rising upward out of the body into 'baramdham'.

5. The Radha Swami Sect Meditation

This group teaches a form of meditation called Suarat Shabd Yoga based on the belief that God is considered to be the Union between Radha (Soul) and Soami (the Master). Basic teachings indicate that initiation for Him comes through a living master so that through the grace of the Guru the disciple can see the light and hear the divine sound. According to this sect the purity of conduct i.e. chastity, vegetarian diet and contact with the Guru are necessary requirements to have the pleasure of His bliss.

6. Buddhist Meditation

Buddhist meditation has its objective of giving ultimate freedom to its performer by quietening the mind whereby all the sufferings, ills, sorrows and their impact gets reduced and this makes way for the spiritual advancement. This stage has been termed as Nirvana which is neither a thing nor a nothing; it is beyond both. This stage consists of the quiescence of all phenomena including speech. As per Lord Buddha there are five obstacles towards the path to spiritual advancement and they are

    (a) sensual desire.

    (b) ill-will.

    (c) sloth and torpor.

    (d) restless ness and worry.

    (e) sceptical doubt.

The four truths which are necessary to be understood are

    (a) truth of suffering.

    (b) truth of the origin of suffering.

    (c) truth of the cessation of suffering, and

    (d) truth of the path leading to the end of suffering.

The groups of clingings for which one must be conscious of, are as follows :

    (a) Investigation of mental objects,

    (b) mindfulness,

(c) energy,

(d) joy,

(e) calm,

(f) concentration and

(g) even-mindedness.

Watchfulness of all the truths, clingings, hindrances are the basic requisites of be observed by a practitioner of this meditation. Awareness to the body, feeling, and mental objects is necessary for attaining nirvana. The Buddha has repeatedly emphasised the need of developing calmness and insight for the extinction of lust, hate and delusion.

The technique of this kind of meditation requires the meditator to sit quietly with spine straight and hands forming a gentle oval. The students try to dissolve their ego, quieten the chattering mind and thereby try to contact the Universal Buddha mind. In this technique the meditators recite nonstop for hours mantra –

Buddham Sharanam Gachami

Dharmam Sharanam Gachami

Sangham Sharanam Gachami

(I take refuge in the Buddha, the Dharma and the Sangha)

The four stages of this meditation which lead one to transquillity are as follows :

1. In the first stage meditator gets aloof from sensuality and sinful thoughts and happiness gets generated by abstraction, reflection and investigation.

2. In the second stage, joy and happiness get generated without reflection and investigation.

3. The third stage is characterized by the even-mindedness through happiness and cessation of passion. It is a stage of equanimity, watchfullness and bliss.

4. The fourth stage is when there is no happiness or misery, joy or sorrow, pleasure or pain. Besides this one is free from inspiration, respiration, reflection and investigation.

7. Zen Meditation

Zen is a Japanese word which means meditation. Its meaning is more like a word intuition and realisation. It indicates a way of life in which there is no difference between internal self and the external world; between thought and action; between unconscious mind and conscious mind. In this kind of meditation one sits in zen motionless posture with straight spine and hands forming a gentle oval. In this process one tries to dissolve the ego, quieten the chattering mind and contact the Universal Buddha mind. The initial stage involves concentration on inhalation (breathing in) and exhalation (breathing out). Then comes the stage of finding solution not through rational process but by self enquiry with full involvement of head and heart. It is placing the problem in such a way that each inquiry goes on clearly in the subconscious mind. Final stage is a time where all actions are done with full attention and awareness. Researches show the results of this meditation are almost similar to yogic meditation.

8. Jiddu Krishnamurthy's Views

It would not be out of context to mention his phlosphy, although Jiddu Krishnamurthy was against any form of planned or structured meditation. According to him meditation is not a search or a probing or a seeking. It is not the taming of the mind to conform, rather it is the total emptiness of mind. He recommends a state of choiceless awareness where the mind is fully occupied by the present moment.

Though all the approaches of meditation adopt different techniques, all of them basically cover purification of mind which has great impact on tension bearing capacity of a person.

HYPNOSIS : A TECHNIQUE OF TENSION REDUCTION

Hypnosis is an important method of experimental psychology which plays a vital role in handling problems created by tension. Auguste Liebeault, a famous researcher in the field of hypnosis, has stated in his research work of 1864 that hypnosis is an extension of suggestability that began by having the subject focus on the idea of sleep. During ensuring of sleep, a suggestion is initiated by the hypnotist and is retained in the conscious level of the subject. This establishes the necessary support and rapport between the subject and the hypnotist.

The famous psychologist Sigmund Freud has observed in his research work that suggestions given during hypnosis often would not be available for the recall after awakening but those forgotten suggestions however could be carried out post hypnotically with a patient rationalizing for his act. Further Freud has concluded in his research work that much of human behaviour is in fact the result of unconscious motivation. It has been observed by researchers in this field that suggestions planted during the hypnotic period have an incredibly strong influence on the subject after the hypnotic period is over. This technique has been found valuable in the treatment of tabacco habit, over eating habits, inferiority-complex etc. As all diseases produce tension, this technique has been found quite useful in removing diseases and the tension they produce.

Some researchers link the effects of hypnosis with trance state while others give a cognitive behavioural explanation. The former category of researchers define hypnosis as a trance state characterized by a very relaxed drowsy and lethargic appearance (Conn & Conn, 1967 ; From & Shor, 1972; Hilgard, 1965; Orns, 1965). In trance state, a hypnotised person loses initiatives to carry out his plan. His energy is diverted from the activity he was engaged towards the instructions of the hypnotist. This has heightened ability to produce fantasies and has an increased susceptibility to suggestion (Hilgard, 1965).

Another definition given by other researchers in this field, says that hypnosis does not include the concept of a trance state but instead it results from positive attitudes, strong motivations and positive enhanced expectancies towards the situation in which the subject finds himself. (Barber, Spance & Chaves, 1974).

The psychologist Josef Breuer discovered that the root causes of hysteric symptoms were painful memories and pent up emotions buried below consciousness. The hysteric symptoms could be eliminated in an indirect manner by encouraging spontaneous verbalisation by patient under hypnosis to evoke a catharsis of the pent up energies causing the symptom.

Employing hypnosis in the treatment of anxiety, Lazarus (1963) has reported that if a patient is asked to simulate a state of sensory deprivation during hypnosis experiences relaxation and calmness. This results in a marked reduction in free floating anxiety. Sensory deprivation may be induced in many different ways. In the strict sense such deprivation involves the elimination of visual, auditory, tactual (touch) olfactory (smell) and gustatory (taste) sources of information for a period of time. Rarely, however, all five senses are restricted.

Simulated deprivation involves the gradual reduction and elimination of sensory information with the aid of hypnotic suggestions e.g. a subject may be told under hypnosis that he is losing all sense of touch. When such a state is induced during hypnosis, a feeling of anxiety is often replaced with a state of calmness.

Reflection of Alpha and Beta Waves During Hypnosis

When a subject has his eyes open and when one is cognitively active, this state is reflected in EEG machines by the presence of beta waves viz machine reflect high frequency, low amplitude waves. Against this if the subject has his eyes closed but nevertheless he is in wakeful position without actively involved in any mental activity, this state is reflected in EEG machine by the presence of alpha waves. It is the state of low frequency and high amplitude. The third state reflected in EEG machine is a state of low amplitude with low frequency which reflect presence of delta waves. Jakobson & Kales (1965) found an absence of delta waves during hypnosis. There is evidence to suggest that alpha wave activity can be altered or manipulated. (Kamiya, 1969), Merininn (1955), found that subjects high in hypnotic suspectability showed decrease in the amplitude and frequency of alpha waves during hypnosis.

The behaviours which result from tension are, inability to concentrate, difficulty in making decisions, extreme sensitivity discouragement, sleep disturbance, excessive sweating and sustained muscle tension. In terms of research works of Coleman, 1976, all the above can be changed with hypnotic suggestions. Motivational level of a person can be changed by hypnosis which can change the behaviour of a person and thereby one can get rid of tension. In hypnosis, enhancement of bodily relaxation can be induced by suggestion. This technique can make the subject visualise pleasant feeling and thereby relaxation is induced into body and mind. This technique has been established as capable of producing many results which are not possible in normal wakeful state.

COGNITIVE THERAPY : FOR REDUCTION OF TENSION

It has been seen that encephalic events contribute to the development and maintenance of pathologic anxiety. Since encephalic events have been learnt and conditioned, they can be unlearnt and deconditioned. Modifying the emotional impact of certain beliefs and perception of visual images and thoughts have been described as cognitive restructuring.

Cognitive therapy is designed to reveal and breakdown irrational belief that leads to distress. In this skill an individual replaces those thoughts which create tension by rational positive thoughts. This is a type of analysis of a situation in which a person develops an insight of the problem and replaces it with rational positive and constructive thoughts which create pleasure. By this technique an individual monitors his own internal arousal level to remain calm and quite in response to provocative situations. This self monitoring is done by adopting any of the following skills through conscious efforts.

(a) **Re-thinking** : This is a technique to substitute constructive ideas to the dead end thought. This helps in allowing one's emotions to subside. It is basically a technique of substituting undesired thoughts with desired ones in a particular situation.

(b) **Stop thinking :** It is a technique to eliminate those ideas which create imbalance resulting in emotional turmoil. By this process one can clear the existing mental state of affairs by blanking of ideas.

(c) **Diversion of mind :** This technique helps in diverting one's mind from the object creating tension to a pleasure giving object.

(d) **Foreseeing a situation :** One can use this technique by foreseeing all the negative points of the situation which are likely to be encountered in the mental framework before the situation actually takes place. This method helps in reducing the level of intensity of the situation which can create emotional imbalance. This is a therapy to increase one's tension bearing capacity.

BIO-FEEDBACK : A TECHNIQUE FOR REDUCTION OF TENSION

Bio-feedback techniques teach an individual to voluntarily control involuntary activity with the use of various instruments. This technique helps in making conscious efforts of a person to modify his internal responses such as heart rate, blood pressure, brain wave creation, certain muscle activity and body temperature by closely observing their effect on bio-feedback machines. The various bio-feedback machines through which visual or auditory feedback comes are as follows :

(a) **E.E.G. :** These machines point out a state of arousal through reflection of brain waves.

(b) **E.M.G. :** These machines tell about muscle tension.

(c) **The temperature feedback machines :** These machines help in knowing flow of blood in different parts of the body.

Researches have established that even involuntary physiological responses could be brought under control through the instrumental conditioning, by watching such responses and making a person conscious of it.

In this technique a person is attached with feedback devices that indicate heart beats and skin temperature. Green light, red light and amber light in this machine respectively indicate whether heart is working slow, fast or within permissible limit.

Bio-feedback is effective as it trains a person in learning the art of relaxation which in turn lowers sympathetic nervous system activity. By this way one can be conscious of bad effects that tension produces.

MUSIC – A TECHNIQUE OF RELAXATION

Music acts as a gateway to bring peace and happiness. By scientific methods it has been proved that music is an important technique of relaxation. Dr Clyde Nash, Jr, of St. Luke Hospital in Cleveland, Ohio, says that music not only helps a patient to relax but also reduces doctor's tension in the operation theatre. The patients who have already undergone operation without music when experienced an operation with music, found it to be a better alternative to anaesthesia. In many hospitals for the treatment of various disorders, music is used with conventional therapy. Studies by music therapist Halen, Lindquist & Bonny suggest that surgery patients experience lower blood pressure and reduce heart rates while treated to soothing-classic music before their operations. Similarly, patients need less pain medication and are able to leave the hospital sooner when exposed to more tunes after their surgeries. A psychologist, Janet Lapp of California State University, concluded that music acts as a better supplemental therapy in comparison to biofeedback and relaxation techniques in the case of patients suffering from migraine-headache. Dr. Oliver Sacks has concluded that music processing is done in the mind by both hemispheres of the brain and play effective role in curing patients suffering from neurological disorders.

Sound comes in circles and one hears it at centre, which is absolute soundless and it produces different effects on a person depending on his liking. Sound that produces pleasing effects helps in creating relaxation of muscles and the mind.

Every music has three phases, i.e.

(a) The meaning of the song.

(b) The laws of music.

(c) The sounds or language of music.

Though in all types of music, all the three phases are necessarily to be there but one can enjoy even taking care of one aspect. Music has been broadly classified into three categories based on gunas that each music involve :

(i) **Sattavic :** This type of music relaxes both singers and audience. Hymnal music which is sung in His praise for His realisation belongs to this category. This type of music is called Nada-Yoga.

(ii) **Raajasic :** In this grade of music all rules of the science of music are rigorously followed by the singers. Such type of music may not be so relaxing but it does not produce any noise pollution and is not jarring to the hearers.

(iii) **Taamsic :** Modern rock'n roll belongs to this category. This type of music creates only momentary pleasure but in long run it creates problems similar to noise pollution.

Music plays a pivotal role in meditation for bringing calmness and creating soothing effect. One is supposed to be alert by becoming conscious of the innermost core of it. This technique of music which was initially developed for creating awareness, is being used for relaxation by way of self-forgetfulness. Music gives short term relief in the form of relaxation by the sound it creates outwardly. When this sound is used inwardly then relaxation takes the form of samadhi which creates long time relaxation of body and mind, and increases tension bearing capacity of a person.

LAUGHTER : A TECHNIQUE OF TENSION REDUCTION

This world is not a tragedy but a comedy. One who has learnt the technique of deep laughter, he has learnt everything. In the words of R.L. Stevenson, "That man is a success who has lived well, laughed often and loved much; who has gained the respect of intelligent men and the love of children; who has filled his niche and accomplished his task; who leaves the world better than he found it whether by an improved poppy, a perfect poem or a reduced soul; who never lacked appreciation of earth's beauty or failed to express it; who looked for the best in others and gave the best he had".

One's emotions speak of one's personality. Our emotions have great impact on the persons around us. Emotions can be positive like laughter, optimism, self-confidence etc., or negative like distress, anger, fear etc. One can increase one's tension bearing capacity by consciously involving his self in positive emotions to the best possible extent. The role of laughter – emotion has got world-wide acceptance for the reduction of tension.

Laughter acts as a powerful drug with no side effects which relieves people from tension of mind and exhaustion of body by injecting new stimulating spirit. By this process one's behaviour and temperament change which leave cheerful personality. Researchers have established that the following changes take place due to laughter :

1. It stimulates production of beta endorphis, a brain chemical which reduces pain and give a feeling of happiness.
2. It acts as a natural pain killer in the body.
3. It improves digestion.
4. It is a good antidote to stress and tones up the system too.
5. Facial muscles, while laughing, instruct the brain to feel good.
6. It increases one's life span.
7. It deepens breathing.
8. It speeds up the process of tissue healing.
9. It improves blood circulation.
10. It stabilises many body functions.
11. It oscilliates immune system.

However it is necessary to remember the precautions that are suggested for laughter.

(a) Don't laugh at others expense or at their disability.
(b) Don't laugh with food in mouth as food may get into

the wind pipe and may result into serious complication.

It has been physiologically established that in smile only seventeen muscles are involved against the involvement of forty muscles in frowning. The important principles of laughter and smile are :

(a) Laugh and the whole world laughs with you, weep and you weep alone.

(b) Smile and somebody some where will smile back at you. Smile is an demonstration of an open attitude to conversation.

It is a fact that many individuals can't laugh at themselves. If one does an introspection, tension bearing capacity of a person can be increased. Osho Rajneesh says: "To me, to laugh wholeheartedly is the greatest celebration that can happen to a man.... to laugh wholeheartedly, to become the laughter. Then no mediation is needed, it is enough." As per Osho, sometimes even great scriptures can't go as deep as a joke can go, because the joke directly touches the heart whereas scripture goes into the intellect. According to Mark Twain the best way to cheer oneself up is to try and cheer somebody else up. As per Swami Ram Tirath, it is the law of nature that action and reaction are opposite and equal.... One can't feel happy unless he has made somebody happy. It has been rightly said that a happy heart is like a balloon which one can't keep down. However, laughter can also be created by any of the three methods mentioned below:

(a) Laughing with mouth shut. In this method one laughs without making sound by keeping the mouth shut, laughing is done internally wherein it is felt that each and every limb of one's body is laughing. This tones up specially intestines.

(b) Laughing with open mouth but without sound. This creates special effect on lungs and digestive system.

(c) Laughing loudly : In this method mouth is kept open, hands are raised to make way for more and more oxygen for lungs and one laughs with sound.

All the three methods tone up the nervous system and increase the tension bearing capacity of a person. The effect that laugh produces can be compared with state when one is in deep meditation. In those few moments of laugh, when thinking process stops, as laugh and thinking are diametrically opposite. The beneficial effects of meditation are bound to enter the body due to the vacuum that is created in the laughing process, which leads to relaxation of body and mind. Laughing is one of the psychological coping and damage repair mechanism built into a human system. It is viewing setbacks and hurts with a sense of humour and trying to joke about it. This pattern both alleviates emotional tension and helps an individual to see the experience in broader perspective. When this mechanism fails the individual bursts into tears.

CRYING AND COPING TENSION

Crying and coping tension is one inbuilt psychological coping and damage repair mechanism that operates in a human body. Crying out is a common means of alleviating emotional tension and hurt feelings. Such reactions can commonly be observed in children. This is one of the means to regain emotional equilibrium and mental poise.

SEEKING SUPPORT

This is another inbuilt psychological coping and damage repair mechanisms that exists in human systems to withstand stress and tension. Seeking emotional support from others till one regains one's own equilibrium is one of the mechanism by which ill-effects of tension can be kept apart and away.

DREAMING AND NIGHTMARES

Dreaming nightmare is coping and damage repair mechanism that exists in human system which operates on a psychological level. It has been seen that individuals who have undergone highly traumatic experiences often report dreams or nightmares in which they get relief of the traumatic experience.

Dreams manifest uncertainty and fear of those unfinished happenings which the dreamer feels are important for subsequent decision in life. It is important to remember that individuals having extreme personalities either strong or feeble, rarely dream because the former category of persons are able to solve most of their problems in conscious state and the latter category of persons on account of the fact that they are not creative either they do not face the problem or don't strive for a solution.

In real life every one faces situation in which one does not find solution during the conscious state. it is necessary to understand the three drives by which one's behaviour is influenced, which are as follows :

(a) Biological Drives (Id).

(b) Social Rules (Super Ego).

(c) Mediating thought processes (Ego).

Id follows the pleasure principle and represents blind demands for instant gratification without caring for social norms and morals. Super ego represents the prohibitive rules and ideals of society which a person is expected to follow. And lastly ego, is basically a mediator between the aforesaid two forces by compromising between the two extremes. In compromising the two extremes, tension takes birth as ego tries to satisfy Id's urges for pleasure within the parameter of social norms. Our behaviour is determined by the instincts and desires that are concealed in one's conscious and unconscious mind thought and behaviour.

A person does his worldly tasks through conscious mind, but unconscious impulses from unconscious mind keep on coming to the conscious mind and affect one's behaviour. At conscious level, one is aware of the things that are around, and at the preconscious levels one is aware of memories and thoughts which can be easily recalled. Against this at unconscious level are the memories, motives and thoughts which cannot be easily recalled.

Id lies entirely in unconscious mind whereas ego and super ego fall in all the three levels of consciousness, (conscious, sub-conscious and unconscious). It is through natural and automatic process that one can repress ideas, memories, motives and feelings which are unacceptable to oneself or which create disturbing result. Such repressed materials, which have not been able to find outlet, do not remain silent and keep on coming to surface level of consciousness and in that process they create disturbed behaviour. Major portion of mind is constituted by this sub-conscious and unconscious mind. The unconscious mind does not know logic and it is more powerful than the conscious mind. These collected emotions and suppressed desires of unconscious mind express themselves in pure or altered forms in awakened or a sleep state. Dreaming is basically a disguised manifestation of Id motives.

ACTING : A TECHNIQUE OF TENSION REDUCTION

Peterbrooh has rightly said "when an actor is inhabited by his role, he really and truly plays his part in totality, one can't see any trace of separation between the him, who is not the role and the him, who is the role, the two are fused completely"

The above quotation itself speaks of the role of acting, actor and the affects of role. Research studies have established that behaving in certain ways can change one's feelings. Mental practice can have the same effect as real practice. Creative researchers have suggested that one can get into happy mood by thinking about a happy period of one's life. Slide into imaging what one wants to achieve, from giving a great speech to hitting a perfect golf shot. Make the experience as real and detailed as one can. Take it from the beginning through successful completion. Latest research of School of Medicine of University of California, in San Francisco, have concluded that every one has got six facial expressions and each signify a specific emotion.

The six emotions are :

1. Surprise
2. Disgust
3. Sadness
4. Anger
5. Fear
6. Happiness

The conclusions of the Californian study suggest that everyone has to do five things to get optimum results in one's life :

(a) Pretend to laugh.

(b) Read with expression and read that conveys a mood other than sadness.

(c) **Relax :** During relaxation there is reduction in heart and breathing rates, consumption of oxygen and blood lactate level goes down.

(d) **Diversion :** This helps in reducing tension when one involves oneself in something stimulating and different e.g. watch movies and divert attention from the source of tension.

(e) Think of one's own positive points to increase selfconfidence. Grooming also helps in gaining self-confidence. For this there is a need to rehearse and tell oneself that one is looking smart.

At last, it is important to remember that one's deeds determine one's image. Thinking can be deceived easily by acting. Recurring acting ultimately emerge as part of behaviour. A therapist can help an individual to see these patterns which in turn help in examining reasons why one continues to choose them. Drama therapy attempts to increase an individual's self-control by providing him with the opportunity and group support to experiment with other more satisfying roles. The desired emotions can be created in body merely by acting and the same technique can be used for increasing tension bearing capacity of a person.

III. PHYSICAL EXERCISE AND TENSION MANAGEMENT

ACROBATICS : A Technique for Tension Reduction

The various types of exercises can be broadly classified as :

1. Body-building exercises.
2. Toning-up exercises.
3. Relaxation exercises.
4. Body shaping exercises.

As per naturopathy, there is a need to conserve vital energy that one possesses. All exercises do not promote real health. There is need to preserve this vital power by its proper use. Life is not supported by body but by the vital power. This approach has emphasised conservation of energy for relaxation which tones up one's system to fight effectively against diseases and thereby increases tension bearing capacity of the person.

In modern life we dislike physical work in all forms and such attitude makes muscles lazy and leads to weakness of the same. If physical exercises are undertaken, we can avoid our blood circulation from becoming sluggish and sluggishness makes a person more prone to tension. One of the best ways to reduce tension is to like and love work. Physical activity if undertaken within permissible limits, increases tension bearing capacity of a person. Aerobic exercises are those which strengthen one's heart, lung capacity and oxygenate the blood. Jogging, swimming, cycling, calisthenic, skipping and even dancing can be acrobatic if performed with this objective in mind.

In tension, one's body chemical undergoes changes in the muscles. Exercise helps in decreasing muscles electric charge and it works like a tranquilizer. Exercise acts as a means through which blocked energy finds outlet and releases tension in a natural way. It helps to learn the technique of tapping the reserve energy, vitality and endurance inside one's self. Exercise keeps depression at bay and controls one's temper. Regular dynamic exercises result in lowering of both systolic and diastolic blood pressure on account of the fact that it results into :

(a) weight reduction,

(b) lowering plasma levels of catecholamines,

(c) increased levels of resodilatory substances like prosta glandins and,

(d) decreased plasma renin activity and blood viscocity.

Regular exercise increases a person's aerobic (oxygen-using) capacity. This increase in aerobic capacity causes a subsequent increase in metabolic rate (how fast one can burn calories). When these exercises are undertaken daily for about half an hour which make use of 75% capacity of lungs then the benefit for the same continues for whole day. Regular exercises help in increasing the working of the various systems of the body thereby leading a person to a healthy life by increasing one's tension bearing capacity.

DANCE

Dance is a physical, mental and spiritual exercise for reduction of tension. All dances speak body language and as such are physically demanding. The prime of all dedicated dances requires emotional discipline and tremendous concentration. Dances like Bharatanatyam and Kathak are not only physical excercises but are almost mental aesthetic yoga. To understand the art of true dance one requires true understanding of life. Dances give a lot of self satisfaction to the performers when the body and soul create full rapport. This stage of performance gives real happiness to its performer and keeps one away from tension. The physical exercise part of dance, helps in removing blockade of energy created by tension. Happy emotions created through acting lead to beneficial effects of dance.

Some dances like Bharatanatyam, get its origin in temple and its irrecoverable identity lies in its spiritual aspects. Dance in itself is like meditation. When dance is taken as meditation, it is movement of body's parts in a natural flow and playing with life energy, bio-energy. Whether we take dance as physical, mental or spiritual exercise it creates beneficial effects in body which increases tension bearing capacity of a person.

SWIMINING

Swimming is an ideal exercise as it engages practically complete range of motions. It helps in toning up the pectoral muscles and support the bust. This tones up the upper arms and makes body more flexible. It cleans, rejuvenates and refreshes the body and thereby increases tension bearing capacity of a person.

AUTOGENIC TRAINING – A Technique of Relaxation

It is a technique which induces abreative emotional discharges. It focuses attention primaril on sensations of diminished sympathetic and increased para sympathetic nervous system activity. This type of training is like giving auto suggestion to become warm and light. Suggestions in this training is given to emotions and breathing, to come from exhalted stage to normal stage.

PROGRESSIVE PHYSICAL RELAXATION – A Technique of Relaxation

This is a technique to activate oneself from the stress response deliberately. By the skill of this technique, stressful response of a situation, is substituted with relaxation response by activating para sympathetic nervous system. In this technique, conscious effort is made to see the effects of various emotions and activities on various organs and systems of the body. The approach of this technique is like bio-feed method whereas feedback is done through bio-feed back machines like ECG, EMG, temperature feedback machines.

Practising this technique in private carries over to enable a person to operate with a lower level of reactivity in social situation. (Benson, 1975).

MASSAGE – A Technique of Relaxation

Massage is an effective measure in increasing the circulation of blood in body and thereby gives relief from fatigue, weakness and pain. A massage often lulls the person involved in massage to go to sleep. It relaxes the body and mind completely. The waste matters which accumulates in the tissues, is got rid of by two ways-one is through veins and other by lymphatic vessels. The purpose of massage is to accelerate elimination process with the help of proper circulation of blood in the veins. As all blood goes to heart for purification it is recommended that the massage should be done in the direction of heart. By this way, working of systems of body get activated and helps in overcoming diseases. This method helps in increasing tension bearing capacity of a person as all diseases produce tension.

SEX – Myth and Reality as a Reliever of Tension

Sex is basically shared experience through physical and emotional union of two persons to have momentary pleasure.

It is a basic urge of all human beings and is a biological need triggered by hormones secreted by glands.

This is a first step for realisation of love which can be realised only when two persons surrender their ego to get merged into one entity. Once this important principle is understood and is expected to merge one's entity with higher self rather than with another entity. For getting this momentary pleasure one wastes lot of energy which otherwise is needed by a human being for carrying out various jobs. The basic reason for even this momentary pleasure is on account of surrender of ego and in these few moments, mind is considered to be empty.

Every disease causes tension. The love-making process reduces tension by improving one's immune system. It strengthens the flow of lymph-fluid throughout the body which helps in removing bacteria, toxins and wastes which build up body tissues. Researches as reported in "The British Journal of Sexual Medicine" show that after love-making one not only drifts off to sleep faster but this prolongs sleep to the extent of 25%. It works as a tranquilizer and promotes relaxation. The sensual massage created during the process of love-making relieves stiffness in muscles. The flow of lymphocytes increases which revitalizes our immune system. It acts as an antidote for nervous tension. Some of the other points that advocate the need to go for love-making are as follows :

(a) It improves blood circulation. This process releases body's endorphins into the blood stream which leave one with a feeling of well being.

(b) It works as one of the antidotes for nervous tension.

(c) It is good for mental health as it brings out strong emotions.

(d) It encourages saliva to wash food from the teeth which lowers the level of the acid that causes decay and prevents plaque to build up.

(e) It burns up calories. In one session of love making 200 to 600 calories get burnt which is equal to 1 ½ hours burning of calories in an exercise with bicycle.

(f) It raises the probability of conception. A book "Mystery, Dance, by Lynn U Margulis and Horion Sagan" cites data which suggest that contraction of the vagina and uterus during climax draw sperm towards the egg which increases the conception chances.

(g) It improves production of hormone estrogen and increases the supply of oxygen which makes hair shine and smoothens skin.

The effects of sex can be classified at three levels :

(a) On psychological level.

(b) On physiological level.

(c) On spiritual level.

The principles learnt from sex should be used on spiritual level where merging is done with inner self which gives a long term pleasure and can act as an instrument and reliever of tension. There is need to have enlightened sexual act which can open gates to samadhi.

Tension is a by-product of energy moving downward. Once this is realised there arises need to conserve vital energy within the body. This conservation of vital energy is possible only through silence, prayer, yoga and meditation. There arises need to transform the basic urge of a human being for a higher cause which is primarily the aim and teaching of all religions. As per Swami Ramtiratha, when marriage is slavery of passion, each time you are satisfied, thraldom is intensified, we sink lower and lower.

Sex is both cause and effect of tension. The general effect of tension is to diminish the overall functioning of male and female sex apparatus. Prolonged stress sharply decreases the level of primary male hormones i.e. testosterone, which directly influence the sex drive. Studies in the area show that men and women who continuously remain under state of anxiety lose interest in sex. According to Kenneth Lamotto (1975) stress apparently slows the production of sperm cells in the male when a man's sex drive is low or may be diminished due to prolonged stress. One is likely to experience occasional impotence, which can be a devastating occurence. This itself produces great emotional disturbance and anxiety for the man, further increasing his stress level.

Research studies also show that important sex hormones in women i.e. progesterone, diminish sharply in women who are constantly in the state of anxiety. Frigidity is a common result of protracted stress and the emotional difficulties usually associated with sexual-dysfunctioning provide the woman with extra obstacles to reduce the tension she feels. Tension plays an important role for creating sexually disordered behaviour e.g. homo-sexuality. An individual under tension leads the individual to the state of dysfunctioning of sexual hormones leading to more homosexual cases and this can commonly be seen in the developed countries. Thus there is a need to understand the myth and the reality about sex. There is a need to rise above sex by conserving energy to experience real happiness.

LYING POSITIONS FOR RELAXATION

The contraction in muscles is termed as tension. Lying position is considered to be the most relaxed position as compared to sitting or standing position as the latter involve contraction of postural muscles which maintain the body upright. In lying position all major parts of the body get relaxation as there is little stretch of muscles and gravitational force is minimum as compared to sitting and standing postures. Lying posture involves minimum expenditure of energy because the pull of gravity on various parts of the body is counter-balanced by the support given by the hard-base of bed to nearly all segments of body. The three lying postures for relaxation that can be categorised are :

1. **Relaxed front-lying posture :** In this posture the face is kept on one side and pillow is kept under the head, under the hips, abdomen and lower ribs and one under the feet.

2. **Half-lying leg raised posture :** In this posture, one lies on the floor and keeps the buttocks close to the side of the bed in such a way that it takes right angle position between position above and under the knee of the leg at the knee position. Full support goes to the lower portion of leg under the knee with foot resting in full at bed. One pillow is kept under the curve of neck. Palms are kept on the sides with upward position. This position helps in taking off waste products from the leg and one can easily go for deep breathing in this posture.

3. **Back lying relaxation postures** : In this posture one lies down on firm base with face and palms up facing upwards. Pillows are placed under head, knee and at the foot to allow greater relaxation to spine.

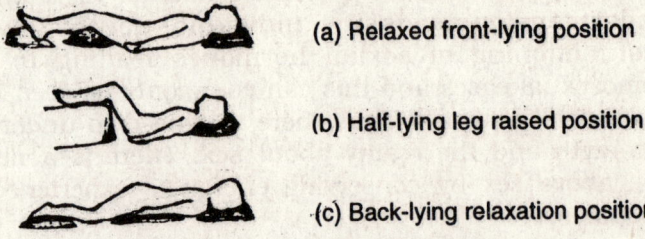

(a) Relaxed front-lying position

(b) Half-lying leg raised position

(c) Back-lying relaxation position

Fig. 6.11 : Relaxed lying positions :

IV. NATUROPATHY AND BIO-MEDICAL THERAPIES

Naturopathy and other bio-medical therapies reflect and constitute the medical approach.

NATURE CURE

All diseases produce tension, it is important to study the various aspects of the system by which a man keeps himself away from tension. Some of the nature cure methods which are effective in keeping a man healthy and free from diseases have been described in the following paragraphs.

1. ACCUPUNCTURE

It is necessary to understand the underlying principles of this Chinese system. According to this philosophy, there exist two types of forces in this universe.

(i) Unifying forces.

(ii) Opposing forces.

The different combination of these forces determine the health of an individual. Medicine is required to correct the imbalance created by opposite forces.

As per this system, it is required to maintain a balance between sympathetic and para-sympathetic divisions of autonomic nervous system. In human body numerous homeostatic mechanisms exist which regulate respiration, heart rate, blood pressure etc. According to this system human body is criss-crossed by a network of pathways called meridians through which life force flows. It is a balance between :

(a) Yin - passive force.

(b) Yang - active force.

When the balance is upset, the meridians get blocked and illness follows. Acupuncture is designed to open-up these blockages. The science consists of inserting the tips of needles into the skin at specific points to stimulate 'nerve' impulses. In human body there are about 2000 acupuncture points and the meridians flow through the organs, nerves, brain, skin and respiration system. Apart from the central and governing meridians there are channels which are bilateral. Yin meridians run from the toes upwards and Yang meridians run from the head and fingertips downwards. Needles, vaccum-cups and gentle thumb massage stimulate flow of lymphatic fluids and release toxins from the muscles.

Accupuncture is considered to be an effective anaesthetic because the needles stimulate the release of endorphins (the brains natural painkillers) and jam the central nervous system which prevents pain signals from reaching the brain. As per this system vital energy flows from channels and organs. By deficiency or blockage of vital energy it is not only the channels or organs but also the preceding and subsequent channels get affected thereby creating diseases. In this process stimulation is done to remove these blockages. It is thus an important system which can be used as effective medium of relaxation. This system helps in increasing body resistance to fight against all infections. It is thus a system which can be used as effective medium for relaxation. It also increases tension bearing capacity of a person by making him more relaxed and disease free.

2. ACCUPRESSURE/REFLEXOLOGY

As per Dr. Fitzgerald, father of this therapy, electric current (chetna), passes through whole body and if any part of the body is not receiving such currents then pain/disease will develop at that point. Switch-boards of these currents for all parts of the body are said to be in two palms and two soles of the feet. As per the principles of this therapy, body can be divided into ten vertical zones running through it like stripes starting from the head and terminating at fingers of hand and toes. All reflex points exist in palms and soles of feet. As this therapy deals with all the reflex points it is called Reflexology. This therapy is also called accupressure because in this technique pressure is given for 10-15 minutes daily at a point for few days to re-charge the electric current of that part of the body where disease is reflected.

As per this therapy, foot massage does relieve tension and is a good treatment for sleeplessness. For nervous tension, this therapy suggests clasping of hands tightly, interlocking the fingers, then with left hand fingers pressed on back side of right hand and then with right hand pressed on the back side of the left hand. The treatment is given for two-three minutes and if repeated for four or five times a day, it helps in overcoming nervous tension. Such treatment, if done for 5-10 minutes at night before going to bed helps ensure good sleep and cure insomnia.

All diseases produce tension and this therapy helps in curing various diseases by making the life current pass in the whole body. This therapy can be said to increase tension-bearing capacity of a person.

3. MAGNETO-THERAPY – A Technique for Reduction of Tension

Magneto-therapy is one of the systems of treatment of various diseases through the application of magnets. Each magnet has two poles, viz north and south. The north pole is believed to kill germs and it stops the development of bacteria. The south pole generates heat and provides energy and warmth to various parts of the body and helps in removing pain and swelling, rigidity and stiffness of any part of body. By this therapy, the functioning of various systems of the body viz circulatory, digestive, nervous, respiratory and urinary can be regulated and controlled, and thereby functioning defects of the body can be reduced. The main principle of magneto-therapy and its advantages are as under :

    (a) Blood veins are spread throughout the body and blood contains haemoglobin which in turn contains elements of iron. By the use of magnet all parts of body can be affected because of the elements of iron.

(b) By the use of magnets over different parts of body, beneficial effect on human metabolism can be produced.

(c) By the use of magnets, blood clotting or clogging can be removed as it makes circulatory system more effective. Use of magnet removes calcium, cholesterol and other deposits from the body and cleans the blood.

(d) The magnetic waves produce heat which helps in removing pain and swelling from the body.

(e) By the use of magnets beneficial effect on the working of autonomic nervous system and internal organs, can be achieved.

(f) By the use of magnets, secretions of hormones can be controlled.

(g) The magnetic treatment works wonderfully in the growth of cells, rejuvenation of tissues and in increasing the number of new blood corpuscles.

(h) This system improves the self-curative faculty, viz homeostasis of the body.

(i) This system removes fatigue and nervousness.

The various beneficial effects that this system produces helps a person to live healthy to enjoy the life by building self confidence and helps in increasing the tension bearing capacity of a person to meet various challenges of the life.

The magnetic treatment has been duly supported by Dr. Hahnemann, the founder of Homeopathy medicine, by the use of whole magnet which is magnetic poliambo and the same covers 397 symptoms. Medicine prepared from north pole covers 459 symptoms. Medicine prepared from south pole is magnet's polus asutrails which covers 387 symptoms. The details of above medicines has been covered by Dr. Hahnemann in his work 'Materia medio' para Vol. II.

4. SPINAL BATH – A Technique for Reduction of Tension

Naturopathy approach emphasises the need to keep the head cool and feet warm to keep oneself healthy. This approach requirs even distribution of body heat to all parts of the body to maintain and improve vitality of the body and mind. This technique produces soothing effect on nervous system and helps in reducing tension. In this, an individual lies down in a tub with head on one side of tub and buttocks on the other side of the tub and feet are kept outside the tub. In this bath, cold water is poured into the tub and the individual remains in the tub for 15 to 30 minutes though adequate care should be taken to cover upper portion of the body with blanket, if the weather so demands.

Spinal bath helps to cool central part of the body, i.e. belly and if it is followed by head bath in which head and face are cooled by pouring cold water for 10-20 minutes. This head bath helps in cooling the brain. Such system of bath acts as health promoting measure for busy executives and helps them to relieve the tension through this method.

5. NATURE CURE THROUGH SNIFFING POWDER

One gram each of coriander seeds, jayphal, black pepper, nausadar (Ammonium Chloride) when grinded and strained through fine cloth to get their uniform mixture and the same is taken as sniffing powder helps in soothing the brain nerves and works as a tonic for tension-reduction.

6. SLEEP

Sleep is a natural device which rejuvenates the whole body to allow it to function more efficiently physiologically during wakefulness. In sound sleep one gets rest and there is direct access to the source of life. It is necessary to know that one spends one third of one's life time in bed for relaxation by way of sleep.

Inadequate sleep has a direct bearing on a person's competence in dealing with stressful situation. Rejuvenation process of sound sleep, has both physiological and psychological effect. This process affects continuously even in dream which apparently relieves one of mental tension, fatigue and stress. In terms of research works of Hattman, (1964), lot of physiological and bio-chemical changes take place during sleep that are believed to allow the body to throw out fatigue and physical tension and stress. Sleep gives rest to our tired muscles and rebuilds body tissues. Its main beneficiary is brain, the most busy and complex part of one's body. It brings a temporary measure of peace by shutting out for a while the mental hubbub of life.

As sleep has a direct bearing on the competence of a person in dealing with stressful situation, it is necessary to understand the basic principles which help in promoting quality sleep to get maximum recouping of energy during sleep.

1. One should go to bed with relaxed body and mind, free from feeling of mental and physical discomforts.

2. One should spend preceding 5-6 hours before sleep in a constructive way which should give happiness and self satisfaction to the person concerned.

An important principle that can be derieved from sleep, is that when one breathes through belly one experiences relaxed state of mind as compared to when one breathes through chest. Tension bearing capacity of a person can be increased by having qualitative sleep. Though sleep can be induced by medicine but it is better to enjoy natural sleep as medicine create its own side effects and benefits of artificial sleep cannot be matched with natural sleep.

7. AUTO-URINE THERAPY

This traditional therapy has been widely discussed over 107 sholakas (verses) in ancient sanskrit in, The Damar Tabtua as expounded by Lord Shiva to his Divine Consort, the Goddess Parvati. As suggested in this book, it is heavenly nectar which is capable of destroying senility and disease.

Dr. Jon Amstrong of America has re-established credibility of auto-urine therapy by his wide spread work in the beginning of this century. The results arrived at after his intensive researches can be summed up as follows :

1. The body begins to absorb more oxygen from the atmosphere after the commencement of auto-urine therapy, and the metabolic reactions are speeded up. The results of a large number of experiments support this conclusion.

2. The commencement of auto-urine therapy is invariably followed by a slow but definite increase in the number of red blood corpuscles in and the haemoglobin content of the blood. Dr. Dharmadhikari believes that these changes in the body functions play a very important part in curing disorders.

In the book 'Yoga' published by the Bihar School of Yoga, Monghyr, a knowledgeable and learned doctor has ascribed the efficacy of urine to the following reasons :

1. Urine supplements the essential nutrients and makes up the deficiency of any nutrient in the body.

2. Urine contains highly active enzymes, that have a salutary effect on all the physiological reactions taking place in the body.

3. Urine contains valuable salts necessary for the body. It has the well-known and widely used twelve salts to cure any and every disease.

4. The hormones contained in urine are of great benefit to the body.

5. Urine possesses bacteriocidal properties. It therefore destroys the disease-causing bacteria in the body especially those infesting the digestive tract.

6. The substances present in the urine augment and sharpen the body's natural powers of resistance to diseases.

7. The substance called 'urea' present in urine is a diuretic and increases the efficiency of the kidneys.

8. Urine is a tonic that strengthens the body, and an 'elixir, that confers longevity.

Ayurveda and other ancient works on medicinal science have accorded their approval to the drinking of urine as a therapeutic measure. Ayurveda regards urine as an effective antidote against harmful confluence of excesses of the three humours.

According to the researches done by the advocates of this therapy, urine consumption promotes the generation of antibodies that helps in overcoming disorders by increasing resistance power in body. Auto-urine therapy helps in overcoming common disorders like colds and coughs, and acute disorders like fever, diarrhoea, vomiting, severe coughs, constipation. It acts powerfully in the disorders of digestive system, respiratory system, genital system, circulatory system and urinary system. Though self-urine is not adviable in disorders such as diabetes, high blood pressure and kidney failure.

BIO-MEDICAL THERAPIES

For tension management there are many bio-medical therapies. Soome these are :

1. BIO-CHEMICAL THERAPY – A Technique for Reduction of Tension

As all diseases produce tension, bio-chemical therapy plays a vital role in reduction of disease and thus this can be called a tension reduction technique. Actually all inorganic substances formed in blood and tissues are sufficient to cure all curable diseases and in a particular way help to regulate constitutional disturbances.

This therapy is based on cell activity and it is necessary to understand that salts which remain after combustion form an essential part of every cell. Bio-chemicals are pure salts homogenous to the cells. Minerals in human body physiologically and chemically are closely related to such salts. With the aid of the minerals, disturbed molecular motions in the cells can be rectified. Such salts help to compensate the losses incurred during a disease. By the use of salts, cells recovery is good and thereby disease is overcome. It has been proved that through special methods of preparations, both mineral and lactose acquire particular physical properties. These salts and minerals when inducted in body cause a disturbance and change the existing state to bring about a restortion of harmony.

Bio-chemical method has been proved very successful in the treatment of constitutional and functional distur-bances, disorders of autonomic nervous system, all types of neuragia, many inflammatory and degenerative processess of all tissues. Against this successful area of treatment, such therapy shows its own limitations. In cases of infections and contagious diseases chemo-therapy and antibiotic treatment has been considered preferable to this method. The twelve mineral substances forming part of theraputic system are :

1. Calcarea floorica (Calc Flur)
2. Calcarea Phosphorica (Calc phos)
3. Ferrum Phospharium (Ferr Phos)
4. Kalium Muriaticm (Kali Mur)
5. Kalium Phospharium (Kali Phos)
6. Kalium Sulffuricum (Kali Sulf)
7. Magnasia Phosphorica (Mag Phos)
8. Natrium Muriatricum (Nat Mur)
9. Natrium Phosphurim (Nat Phos)
10. Natrium Sulfrise (Nat Sulf)
11. Salicea
12. Calcarea Sulphonica (Calc Sulf)

This bio-chemical therapy goes a long way in increasing the tension bearing capacity of a person by reduction or elimination of diseases.

2. HERBAL THERAPY – A Therapy for Reduction of Tension

Ayurvedic approach recognises that all diseases and abnormalties are due to three doshas (disorders) :

(a) Vital Airs,
(b) Bile,
(c) Phlegm.

Herbal therapy emphasises the intake of various herbs to keep the various parts, systems of body in healthy position. As all diseases produce tension, it is necessary to study such therapy to keep oneself healthy and away from disease.

3. ELECTRO SHOCK THERAPY – A Technique for Reduction of Tension and Severe Depression

In this therapy a full body seizure or convulsion is triggered by a quick jolt of electric current. Electrodes are attached to one or both temples and electricity is directly passed through brain which makes patient loose his consciousness. Basic principle behind this therapy is that it increases the availability of certain neurotransmitters in a region of the brain called the limbic system. Electricity enhances feeling of well being by producing 'Cortial Organism'. 'It has been observed that such electro-convulsive shocks can result in producing dizziness and loss of appetite and short term memory loss in some cases.

4. PSYCHOSURGERY

This technique for reduction of tension has been stopped due to availability of latest researches in the form of medicine as post surgery effect produce serious consequences which make the patient dull, aqthetic and drain off emotions and motivations, which are very necessary for a person to live.

The psychosurgery involves removal of brain tissues from profontal cortex from the rest of the brain. It is profontal cortex which is inter-connected with visual and auditory and somato-sesory cortica areas etc. This removal of connections gives permanent solutions to a man but makes a man lifeless.

5. CHEMO THERAPY – A Therapy for Reduction of Tension

This type of therapy in the form of medicines, i.e. chemical substances is most commonly used due to its cheap availability. These chemical substances help in removing the characters of disorders which make a man to feel better. This type of artificiality gives temporary relief to its taker but normally produces side effects which are harmful. Such therapy helps in calming one's nerves, helps oneself to sleep and to brighten one's moods. Drugs which produce tranqualizing effects, reduce tension by soothing the nerves and by this process one can improve upon his social behaviour and sleep patterns which may be shortlived.

V. MISCELLANEOUS THERAPIES

There are some interesting and imaginative therapies which need a special mention. Recreation, aroma, colour, helitherapy and gems have been described here.

RECREATION

Leisure time is very important for increasing relaxation both of body and mind. It gives opportunity for developing and exploring one's interest to understand one's ownself. Free time if utilised properly by way of meaningful and enjoyable activities, it can become source of happiness as it induces relaxation but if free time is taken as free time it can become a cause of tension. Leisure is free time but that must not be forced upon like the time of unemployment or compulsory retirement.

Recreation can be done through finding leisure time which has the following functions :

(a) Rest and refreshment

(b) Entertainment and amusement to compensate for dullness and monotony.

(c) It is enrichment and development of interest and aspects of one's personality which otherwise never find expression. and satiation.

Leisure behaviour is not dependent on personal factors like one's need, interest and ability but also on one's social factors, like position and role in various groups and the standards one has to adhere to, in the given environment.

AROMA THERAPY

Aroma therapy emphasises that smell produces effects on mood, body and mind. The systematic use of it can bring change in life by alleviating stress and tension. The tools of aroma therapy are botanical essences and vegetable oils. Essential oils that are used in this therapy, are extracted from plants and these have direct effect on the body, nervous system and mind. Massage of these oils relaxes tight muscles, open blocked nerves, increase lympth flow and circulation of blood. These massages produce stimulation to the brain which relaxes the body and mind.

Scientific researches have confirmed that essential oils massages and even the smell of them has the power to alter one's state of mind. It can produce beneficial results in the cure of physical, mental and psychosomatic stress problems. The use of these essential oils can be made through a variety of ways including direct inhalation or as a massage. Room freshners and mood enhancers available in market are based on this therapy. Researchers have revealed that smelling of different plants produces different results as follows :

(a) Rose fragrance helps in alleviating hangovers and it produces soothing effect on stress and depression.

(b) Orange plant smell mitigate anxiety, insomnia and worry.

(c) Basil (Tulsi), Rosemary (an evergreen fragrant shrub), Patchouli fragrance stimulate mental clarity, concentration and memory.

Smells of some plants have theraputic and preventive effects and help in overcoming bad effects of various diseases. Eucalyptus has excellent anti-septical and anti-bacterial properties which help an individual to fight with infection and lead a happy healthy life.

COLOUR THERAPY

It has been scientifically established through researches that colours can trigger off many symptoms of tension and can be useful in treatment of mentaly ill patients. Colours have an important role to play in influencing people and their attitude. Our ancients sages knew the importance of colours in healing. Russians proved scientifically that man could feel colours through the skin and that skin is indefinitely more sensitive to sensations than one could have ever thought of. Each colour creates a specific atmosphere and that influences a person's mind.

(a) *Yellow* is the brightest primary colour nearest to sunlight and most luminious. It consequently has cheering effect.

(b) *Red* is most aggressive and demanding colour in the whole spectrum. This colour forces itself on a person. It is used widely for danger signals. It has sexually suggestive quality.

(c) *Orange* is stimulating and psychological tests have shown that if it is used extensively in a room, the occupants feel driven out by its sheer forcefulness.

(d) *Green* is the colour of the nature and is well known for its restful effect on the eyes. It is opposite to red and produces positive sedative.

(e) *Purple* stimulates the brains. It is associate with grandness, royalty and ceremonials.

(f) *Brown* is restful and if used in harmony with another warm colour can take for a cosy setting.

(g) **Blue** has the effect of retreating and is also sedative. Traditionally it is associated with chill of holiness.

Colours can be dingy colours, violent colours and clashing colours. Colours by making change in external environment can act as a powerful therapy for tension reduction.

HELITHERAPY - Therapy through Sun Rays for Reduction of Tension

Various diseases can be cured through this therapy and the tension bearing capacity of a person can be thus increased. Seven colours found in sun rays are red, yellow, orange, blue, green, indigo and violet. In terms of results of various researches, different colours produce different effects on the body. Some of the effects linked with various colours can be summarised as follows :

Orange colour of sun rays : This colour of sun rays produces beneficial effects on stomach, liver, kidney, bronchitis, blood circulation etc. It makes veins stronger and reduces their contraction. It improves brain functioning, it develops courage and inspires a man to gain greater heights in all fields. The problem of excess urination, pain in joints and chest pain can also be overcome by the use of this colour of sun rays.

Green colour of sun rays : This is basically combination of yellow and blue colour. It purifies blood. It improves eliminating functions of the body.

Blue colour of sun rays : This colour produces cooling and soothing effect. It has beneficial effect on throat, is anticeptic and helps in concentration and meditation. It reduces stimulated emotions and high blood pressure. It is good in reducing swelling of different parts of body, arrest the falling of hair, helps in producing sound sleep and healing of burn wound at any portion of body. Different colours produce different artificial minerals which are summarised as follows:

Orange colour has in it : Alkaline, iron, copper, calcium, hydrogen, carbon, barium, arsenic, nickel and aluminium.

Blue colour has in it : Barium, aluminum, lead, copper, oxygen, tin, zinc and phospherus.

Different colours are capable of curing diseases due to the fact that each colour produces different minerals which in turn increases tension bearing capacity of a person.

(a) Passionate   - Purple
(b) Devilish   - Black
(c) Virginal   - White
(d) Blasphemous   - Blue
(e) Scandalous   - Red

At present various colours are available in the market. By proper combination of shades and tints proper atmosphere can be created which has pleasing effect on body and by this therapy tension can be kept apart by change in working environment. Colours play an important role in grooming and creating self confidence. By this confidence, many tense situations can be changed. Colours not only play important role in external environment but help in diagnosing the various types of diseases that a person is suffering by looking at the colour of various parts of the body as follows :

1. Colour of skin shows essence of lungs.
2. Colour of lips shows the essence of spleen.
3. Colour of tongue shows conditions of heart and digestive system.
4. Colour of nails shows the esence of liver.
5. Colour of ears shows essence of kidneys.

It is necessary while making diagnosis that all features be taken together as the body acts as an organic whole. In a nutshell, helitherapy plays a vital role in creating relaxation by making change in external environment and thereby acts as a powerful therapy of tension reduction.

SILENCE AND PATIENCE : Technique of Tension Reduction

By observing silence and patience one can save vital energy which increases one's tension bearing capacity. The process of observing silence helps in setting down thinking process and thereby helps in reducing tension. Silence and patience are powerful tools in breaking the vicious circle of tension. As tension results in change in behaviours and emotions, this has a direct bearing on persons and environment that exist around tense persons. Silence helps in making rational decisions as a person in tension cannot be expected to make rational decisions in the state of disturbed mind.

It has been rightly said that one who can't sensibly control a moment of annoyance, will have to spend days in annoyance. Silence is an important technique to control the string of life. By having control on emotions one can prove the well known quotation "My life is in the hands of any fool who makes me lose my temper".

GEMS THERAPY

This therapy establishes that different gems of different colours produce different beneficial effects and each gem represents its own corresponding star. As in Indian philosophy astrology has its own role to play, The outcome of any endeavour is based on the position of different stars. by using various gems, stars can be effected. Based on this theory the relationship of stars, gems and colours can broadly be summarised as given in Table 6.1 :

Table 6.1

Star	Gem	Colour
Sun	Ruby	Red
Moon	Pearl	Orange
Mars (mangal)	Coral (Moonga)	Yellow
Mercury (Budh)	Emerals (Panna)	Green
Jupiter (Vanaspathi)	Moonstone	Blue
Venus (Sukra)	Diamond	Indigo (Aasman)
Saturn (Shani)	Suppohire (Neelam)	Violet (baggani)
Rahu	Sardinium (Gomdhak)	Deep Violet
Ketu	Cats eyes (lehsunia)	Infrared

As all diseases produce tension, gem therapy believes that by wearing different stones in the form of rings or by placing such gems on chest by wearing mala around neck one can influence the stars. This therapy believes that by wearing such stones the effects that different stars produce can be altered and thereby diseases can be cured.

7

YOGA AND TENSION MANAGEMENT

Yoga is a Sanskrit word derived from the root "Yuj" which means "to join". The process of joining is neither physical nor chemical. The process is so subtle and super fine that when once this joining is complete the man loses one's own entity completely and becomes one with God. Yoga is the conscious and directed activity of an individual aspiring to a supra-sensory and supra-intellectual experience which is to one of spiritual value and which fully or to some extent transforms or deepens one's life and his knowledge or understanding of reality and of oneself. In other words, the aim and purpose of yoga is to bring about a higher and more accomplished state of mind which transcends man's usual and every day experience and opens for one a new field of vision and the capacity to grasp that vision. The whole personality is transformed and can function in a new dimension hitherto unknown or inaccessible to it. Knowledge is widened, deepened and increased and there is a sense of communication with the Infinite or with reality as a whole. Once the link with that vital force is established the individual is no longer cut off from the whole.

Yogasanas have edge over the physical exercises like wrestling, gymnastics etc. Firstly yogasanas have a direct impact on the internal organs whereas other exercises only affect the muscles outwardly and thus on apparent look the latter may show better results but in real sense real health is built with healthy internal organs. Secondly yogasana is effective cleaning process which make functioning of the body more efficient by throwing all wastes of the body. Number of cells that are formed in asanas are larger in number as compared to the cells that are breaked during the process of asanas. Thirdly yogasanas increases elasticity of one's body, normalises one's blood pressure which make one look younger whereas other exercises make muscles stiff and hard which pave for early old age. Fourthly Pranayama expansion and contraction of lungs take place and in this process blood get purified as oxygen reaches innermost portion of lungs. Fifthly by yogasanas, flexibility is brought in spine which controls entire nervous system and blood cirulation system. Sixthly yogasanas are systematic as it makes correct blend of stretching and relaxation of muscles and thus it don't make feel tired after its practice.

Patanjali, the father of yoga, has suggested the following steps which from part of yoga to liberate man from sorrow and to obtain desired physical and mental levels :

1. **Yamas :** Control and discipline (Restraint). It is self restraint through Ahinsa, Satya (truthfulness), Astets, Brahmachariya and Aparigraha (non covetousness).

2. **Niyamas :** Rules, methods and principles (observance). They are Shaucha (purity), Santosha (contentment), Tapa, Swadhyja.

3. **Asanas :** Making body postures.

4. **Pranayama :** Controlling the normal breathing cycle in order to get control over prana, the vital force.

5. **Prathyahara :** The withdrawal of the senses from their respective outside objects and projecting them inwards. It is revolving the matter in the mind in order to understand it.

6. **Dharana :** Concentration, fixing one's mind on an external object.

7. **Dhayana :** Meditating with constant attention on the object of concentration.

8. **Smadhi :** Contemplation, when the mind becomes one with the form of the object of its concentration in dhyana.

In order to facilitate the practitioners, these steps were later grouped under different yogas according to their nature and substance :

Jnana Yoga covers Yama and Niyama,

Hatha Yoga covers Asanas and Pranayamas,

Karma Yoga covers Pratyahara,

Raja Yoga covers Dharma, Dhyana and Samadhi.

Jnana Yoga : It is a science of acquiring proper knowledge. It covers all those areas of nature, society and the self, whose knowledge is essential for warding off sorrow and maintaining a healthy and happy life. It is a realization of a man's own divinity through knowledge.

Karma Yoga : It teaches how to avoid undesirable elements in various actions of an individual and how to act so that a satisfactory result is obtained. It is a manner in which man realise his own divinity through work and duty.

Hatha Yoga : It is primarily concerned with bodily postures– a technique with air, physical excellence but practise of this is important for creating good impact on mental health as well.

Raja Yoga : It is a science of mental excellence. It implies a complete masterry of the self. Raja Yoga and Hatha Yoga form complement to each other and form a single approach toward liberation. The basic three steps are Concentration, Meditation and Contemplation. It is realization of divinity through control of mind.

According to Yoga Science an individual is supreme. He is powerful being. He possesses all the powers himself if he knows how to use his own powers properly, he can obtain what he desires. He alone is the maker of his fate and destiny. The basic yogic theme about an individual and one's inherent powers can be summarised as follows :

(i) Everyone is responsible for what one is today and what one will be tomorrow.

(ii) One is as good as anyone borne in the past or living at present.

(iii) Everyone possess physical and mental powers both of which can be developed and increased.

(iv) Fulfilment of one's desire depends upon one's own actions and thoughts.

(v) One can change oneself.

According to yogic view, spine is comprised of three basic channels which are as follows :

1. IDA nadi starts from left nostril and it is called a nadi of moon.

2. PINGALA nadi starts from right nostril and it is called a nadi of sun.

3. SUSHUMNA is in the middle of Ida and Pingala nadi and hence is called channel of equilibrium. It is the main channel of nervous energy and is situated inside the spinal column.

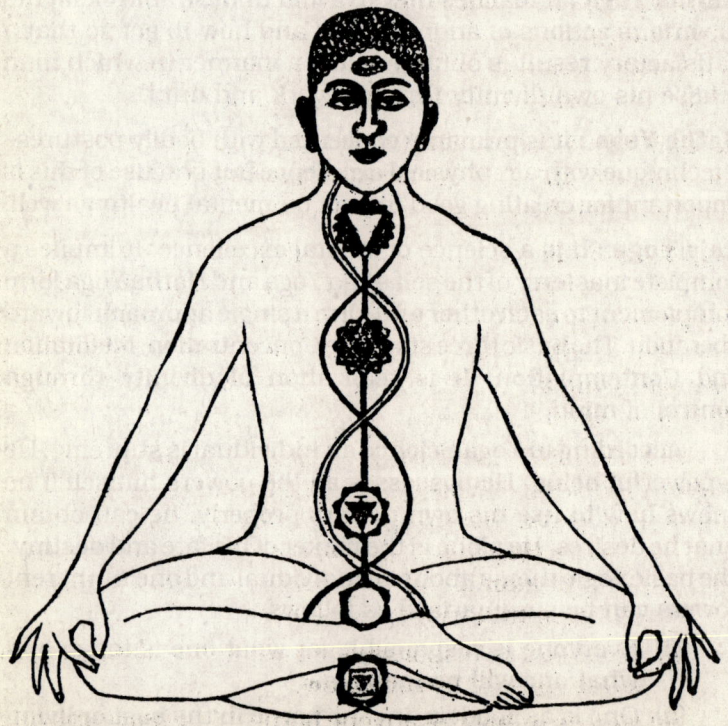

Fig. 7.1 : The nadis Ida and Pingala interwine and coil around Sushuma like the two serpents.

All the above three channels of energy are tapped through –

    (a) Asana,

    (b) Pranayama,

    (c) Bandha,

    (d) Mudra and

    (e) Through other discipline control the basic force is believed to be generated from Mudra where anus and gentals meet which moves upward through sushumna nerve channel to the saharrar.

(a) **Asanas :** Based on certain definite scientific principles, some of the yogic exercises twist the body forward, others help the lateral movements of the spine, yet others keep the thyroid in a healthy condition and supply abundant blood to the brain, and seek to develop the diaphragm and the muscular partition between the chest and abdomen. The western systems of physical exercises develop the superficial muscles of the body. It is left to yogic exercises to exercise thoroughly the internal organs such as the liver, spleen, pancreas, intestines, heart, lungs, brain and the important ductless glands of the body. Some of the asanas promote digestion and circulation of the blood and make the kidneys, liver and all other internal viscera work efficiently. The ancient Rishies of India have formulated these Yoga Asanas not only because they preserved a high standard of health, vigour and vitality in the practitioner but also aid in their moral development and spiritual attainments.

The Need of Asanas

    (a) To improve health.

    (b) To maintain health.

    (c) To cure certain types of pain in the body/back.

    (d) To overcome tiredness.

    (e) To increase the resistance to cold and minor ills.

    (f) To keep and improve the shape of the body.

    (g) To mitigate the strain and tensions of modern living.

(h) To increase vitality and promote a feeling of well being.

(i) To improve the circulation of blood.

Asanas can cure flabby thighs, building waistline, sagging stomach. A series of exercises (asanas) are said to isolate the mind by freezing it from attention to bodily functions. As one gets older, one's muscles tend to get shorter and harder. With this contraction, come loss of activity, extra weight or flabbiness, stiffness, wrinkles, aches and pains which in turn create tension. All this can be avoided by asanas which keep the muscles stretched strong and supple.

"An ounce of practice is better than tons of theory", says Vivekanand. This is true for realisation of real self through the purification of body and mind. Some of the asanas which help in reducing tension by reconditioning of body and mind are as follows :

SHAVASANA

Posture : One is required to lie down with the back on the ground in a relaxed state, facing the sky, eyes closed. One concentrates on the breath.

By doing Shavasana the frequency and intensity of both proprioceptive and denteroceptive impulses in the person gets reduced. This helps the practitioner to become introverts and withdraw from outside world.

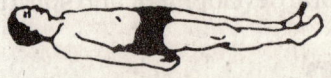

Fig. 7.2 : Shavasana.

It is fact that hypothalamus is the locus of the mind where thinking process for an individual takes place. When the mind has thoughts of worry, the inner harmony gets disturbed and this itself becomes cause for the disturbing various muscles of endocrine glands, harmonal balance, and autonomic nervous system.

Benefits : During Shavasana, mechanism of hypothalamus goes slow which reduces the blood pressure. In this process one is away from tension. This reduces proprioceptive impulses and this relaxes body muscles.

YOG-NINDRA – A technique for Relaxation

Posture : Yog-nindra can be considered to be the next stage of Shavasana as it leads the mind into different layers of consciousness. Shavasana is considered adequate if undertaken for five to fifteen minutes whereas Yog-nindra is required to be undertaken for minimum ten minutes and may be extended to an hour. In Yog-nindra, one is required to lie down with back on ground, hands and legs also on ground in a relaxed state, eyes closed, a pose similar to Shavasana. In this technique a sense of deprivation is created by stopping all messages from all senses to enter the body, concentration is done on breathing and each breath is consciously taken in and out. In each breath constructive suggestion is given to mind by consciously thinking that all diseases are going out of the body. After this conscious effort is made, it is necessary to look into the state of affairs of each part of body and relaxation is induced by conscious effort through constructive ideas. In last stage an effortless approach is made to make oneself alert towards outside realities and atmosphere. After this eyes are opened and a thoughtless stage is induced. The practice of Yog-nindra for a long period of time helps in bringing relaxation to an individual and thereby tension bearing capacity of a person gets drastically increased.

Benefits : Yog-nindra helps in calming down of mind, slowing down of heart beat, less consumption of oxygen, lowering of blood pressure, increase in alpha waves and thereby relaxation of mind is achieved. It is a technique in which conscious effort is made to relax each part of body and thereby muscular, mental and emotional relaxation is induced. Yog-nindra is a stage which lies between full sleep and active awakened mind. It produces better effects of the effects that sleep produces.

SHITHLASANA

Posture : In this asana, one lies down on one's stomach, with face towards right direction by resting left side of face on the ground. Right arm is bent from the elbow so that palm and

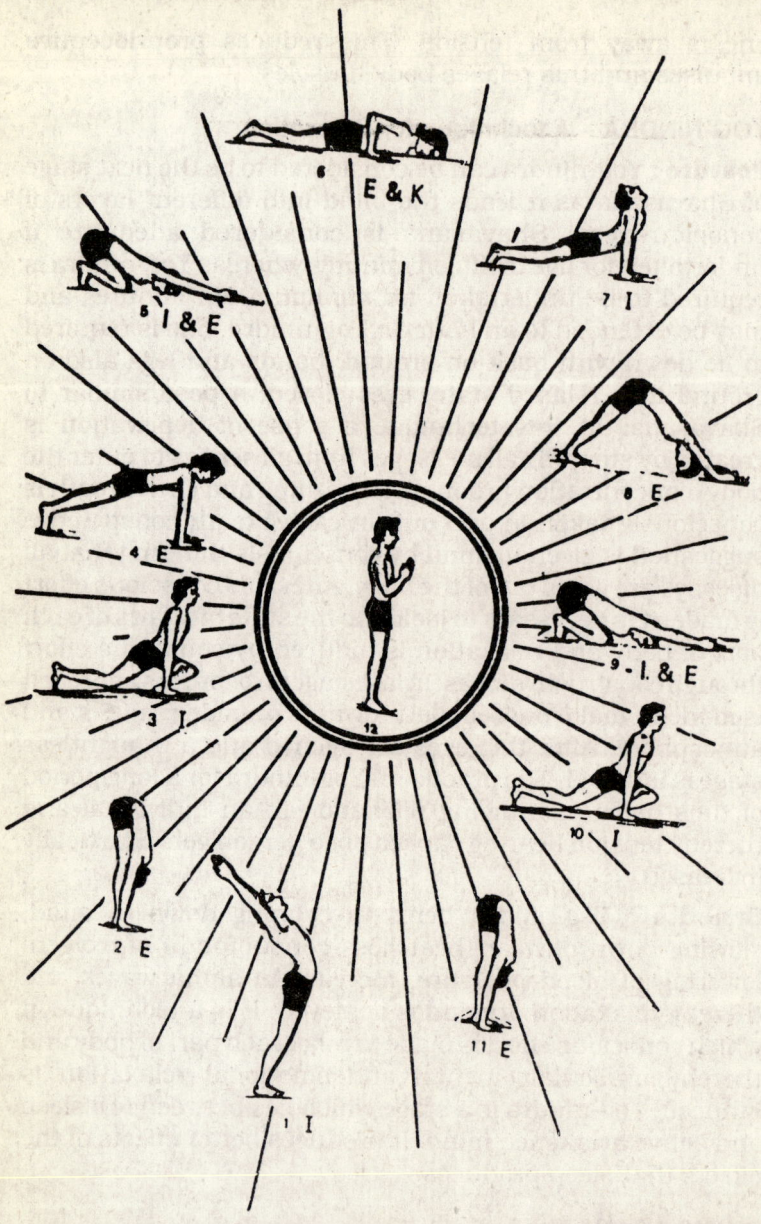

I - Inhalation   E - Exhalation   E & K - Exhale and hold breat

Fig. 7.3 : Suryanamaskar.

fingers of right hand rest on the ground at about 15 cm away from nose. Left arm lie straight. Right leg is bent in such a way that the right foot heel comes near the left leg knee. In this, entire belly and chest touches the ground and the whole body is left loose in a relaxed state. Deep breathing is done during this pose. The above posture is repeated on the other side by keeping right leg and right hand straight. Left leg and left arm are bent as stated above.

Benefit : The asana produces very good results in generating sound sleep and for creating relaxation in body by controlling the thought process. When mind withdraws itself from adverse outer environment and attention goes towards inner self, then one gets peace, enjoy the calmness and tranquility. This process is called meditation in Raj Yoga.

SURYANAMASKAR

Posture : This asana consists of 12 steps required to be done with systematic breathing system of inhaling and exhaling. *Step one* consists of standing pose with folded hands near chest with breath out. *Second step* consists of taking the arms up vertical to body, bending backward with breath in. *Third step* consists of lowering the upper portion, touching the ground with hands facing the knees, this is done with breath out. *Fourth step* consists of keeping one leg between two hands which rest on ground, the other leg is stretched out in full length, upper body is bent towards back, with eyes towards sky. This is done in inhaling stage. *Fifth step* is done with hands touching the ground, mid-portion of the body stretched up with face down to ground and then placing body pressure towards the side. This is done in holding the breath inside. *Sixth step* is done in breathing out with body going to touch the ground with pressure on hands, body weight on ground. *Seventh step* takes Bhoojang Asana pose. Thereafter 5th, 4th, 3rd, 2nd and 1st step are repeated so as to make 8th, 9th, 10th, 11th and 12th step respectively.

Benefits : Suryanamaskar reduces both physical and mental tension. This asana–

(a) Steps up cardiac activity.

(b) Improves the flow of blood throughout the body.

(c) Tones up the nervous system by successively stretching the spinal columns. The functioning of para-sympathetic and sympathetic nervous system becomes more acute.

(d) Ventilates the lungs, oxygenates the blood and acts as a disintoxicant by getting rid of carbon dioxide and other toxic gases through the respiratory tracts.

(e) Stimulates and normalizes the activity of the endocrine gland.

This asana has other beneficial effects on skin, shoulders, neck, wrists, thighs, ankles, abdominal muscles etc. This asana is very effective as it always checks worry and calms down anxiety.

PASCHIMOTTAN ASANA

Posture : In this asana one sits on the floor stretching out both the legs in front and keeping the heels and toes together. Spine, neck and head are kept erect. Then breath is consciously taken in and hands go up and then slowly bend down while exhaling and head is buried in between the knees, the elbows are kept on ground and hands hold the thumbs of the feet.

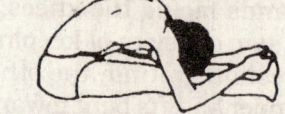

Fig. 7.4 : Pashchimottan Asana.

Benefits : This asana normalises the functioning of nervous system and thereby it has a good conditioning effect on the mind. Its other benefits include in removing the disorders of spine, kidneys, liver and spleen. It helps in strengthening Sushumna nadi. This pose helps in rousing spiritual forces which normally lie dormant at the base of spine.

HALASANA

Posture : In this, one first lies down on the back and stretches one's body. Arms are rested on the sides with palms facing the ground. Then one lifts the legs slowly by placing pressure on the hands by making 90 degree angle, bending the waist by way of half circle, legs are taken beyond the head till feet touch the ground.

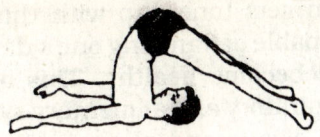

Fig. 7.5 : Halasana.

Benefits : This asana is useful in reducing tension as it is very effective in increasing mental and physical energy. It provides fresh blood to the spine and its ligaments. It has beneficial effects on liver, pancreas, spleen and kidneys.

SARVANGASANA

Posture : In this asana one lie down on the back with hands' palms touches the ground on the sides of the thighs which are resting on the ground. One slowly raises one's legs by placing pressure on one's hands, staying for a while at 45 degree position and bringing them to 90 degrees and stay for a few moments. Then one raise one's waist also and take the legs beyond one's head by bringing legs parallel to the ground. Here one exhale, and start lifting the hands from the ground bending the arms from the elbows, placing hands on the back for proper support. We raises the legs upwards with the elbows resting on the ground. Here the normal breathing takes place.

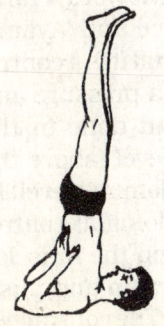

Fig. 7.6 : Sarvangasana.

Benefits : This asana is very useful in reducing tension. As the name suggests, it gives strength to all parts of body. Nervous system gets toned up with this asana, makes a person more capable of handling one's day to day problems. Thyroid glands become healthy. This asana strengthens circulatory, respiratory and ailmentary systems of the body, it makes spine elastic and removes disorders of thyroid, tonsils, neck, lungs and ears.

PRANAYAM AND TENSION

Pranayam is a purification technique of mind which helps in strengthening nervous system, memory and concentration power. It affects beneficially liver, stomach, kidneys, digestive organs etc. Pranayama is control of breathing to rejuvenate the physical body. It stabilizes the rhythm of breathing in order to encourage complete respiratory action. Pranayama when practiced regularly helps one to have control over one's sense organs and the mind. Manu has rightly said "just as the impurities of metals (gold etc.) are removed by the flame of fire, the indriyas (senses) throw out their impurities through Pranayam".

It has been scientifically found that pranayam creates beneficial effects on emotions as there is a deep relationship between emotions and breathing. By controlling one's emotions one can get rid of tension. Pranayama literally consists of Prana and Ayama. The Sanskrit word 'Prana' means 'life' or vital force and 'Ayama' means control, i.e. in total it is a control of Prana. In pranayama pressure and release of pressure and done in the trunk at the thoracic level (above the diaphragm) are the abdominal level. In breathing with the abdominal control there is struggle between the muscles which lower the diaphragm and push the organs downwards. The contracted

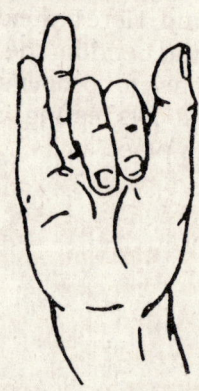

Fig. 7.7 : The Mudra - the mode of holding the right hand fingers for the practice of Pranayama.

abdominal wall is pushed forward which resists that pressure instead of yielding to it. This results in intra-abdominal pressure which produces benefical effects.

Pranayam plays a vital role and effects different parts of the sytem which in turn perform different functions of the body. Pranayama do functions of the body though it has been given different names for the purpose of identification of force;

1. It circulates in the area around the heart and central breathing (Prana).
2. It circulates in the lower region of the abdomen and controls excretory functions. (Apana).
3. It stimulates the gastric juices and aids digestion (Somana).
4. It remains in the thorartic cage and controls the absorption of air and food (Udana).
5. It spreads throughout the body and distributes the energy from food and breath (Vyana).
6. It relieves abdominal pressure by provoking erciation (Naga).
7. It controls the eyelids so as to prevent foreign bodies from entering the dazzling light from harming the eyes (Kurma).
8. It prevents certain substances from rising into the nasal cavities or descending into the throat causing sneezing and coughing (Krkara).
9. It ensures the absorption of extra oxygen into a tired body and causes yawning (Devodutta).
10. It remains in the body even after death and sometimes causes the body to swell (Dhanajaya).

Any imbalances in the functioning of any of the points mentioned above is likely to produce tension of various degrees. The art of Pranayam teaches one to limb up the ladder of mental peace. Pranayama restores calm and equipoise of the disturbed mind and helps in restoring self confidence. Emotional excitement effects the rate of breathing and conversely deliberate regulation of breathing checks emotional excitement which helps in controlling tension. The process of disciplined breathing acts on one's tangled and inchoate nervous system and produces miraculous effect just as rubbing is a bar moecules over an ordinary piece of steel polarises its mollecules and creates a new power in it.

How Does Deep Breathing Help ?

If one increases the volume of intake of air in one's breathing, it has a very benefical effect. This volume of air, to be specific, is a combination of various ingredients e.g. oxygen, nitrogen, moisture, pollutants etc. and it is actually measured as tidal volume. In normal breathing one intakes about 500 ml (millilitre) of air, out of which 150 ml goes waste. If breath intake is increased by fast breathing, the intake of tidal volume 170 ml/minute and against this if one takes deep breathing as is being done in yoga Pranayama, the intake of tidal volume is 1000 ml/minute. By this process, lungs get a lot of oxygen which purifies blood and makes the system more effective thereby increasing one's tension bearing capacity.

It has been scientifically established that there is a close link between emotions and breathings. It is observed that the breathing changes its rate and style under different emotions that man produces. Pranayama plays an important role in changing breath quality that is bound to create positive emotions.

To get a complete picture that Pranayamas effects produces, it is necessary to understand that yogic breathing combines the following three different forms of breathing.

(a) **Diaphragmatic breathing :** According to this process the base of lungs is filled with air and rhythmic lowering of the diaphragm helps the organs of the body to function normally. Diaphragm is basically a strong position of muscles separating the chest and the abdomen.

(b) **The Intercostal breathing :** It helps in filling the middle section of the lungs which allows the fresh air to enter in abdominal respiration. This process is done by raising the ribs through dialation of the thoracic cage or chest wall.

(c) **The Chavucular breathing :** It provides fresh air to upper section of the lungs. This process is done by raising the collar bone and shoulders.

One breathes through both left and right nostril. The flow of prana through the left nostril is done by Ida or Chandra Nadi, which brings cooling effect and influences the left part of the body and controls human thoughts. It has Tamas Guna. The flow of prana through the right nostril is done by Pingala or Surya Nadi. It controls the right part of the body and rings heat producing warm effect. It is supposed to have Rajas Guna. The objective of Pranayama is to bring proper balance between Ida and Pingala for the purpose of attaining spiritual attainment through Susukshmna. Balance between the three Nadis gives strength, health and peace.

Pranayama is different from normal breathing as it is a specific way of inhaling and exhaling. The three ways of controlling breath in Pranayama are :

1. Pooraka – filling the breath.
2. Rechaka – throwing the breath-out.
3. Khumbaka - holding the breath in or out. Holding in the breath is Antrik Khumbaka and holding it after throwing breath is Balya Khumbaka.

The different Pranayamas suggested below are basically different combinations of Pooraka, Rechaka, and Kumbhka,

1. Shawans-presha Pranayama

(a) In this pranayama each breath is consciously inhaled and exhaled with closed eyes. When this is done for a long time, it helps in overcoming tension.

2. Chandra-bhedi Pranayama

In this pranayama, inhaling is done from left nostril and exhaling is done through right nostril. If this type of inhaling and exhaling is combined with closure of hearing and concentration is done on an internal buzzing sound of any type, then it becomes very beneficial in overcoming tension and helps in subsiding aroused emotions.

3. Bhramari Pranayama

In this type of pranayama, ears and eyes are closed with fingers keeping the palms of the hands open. After inhaling fresh air, breath is retained for a few seconds inside by doing

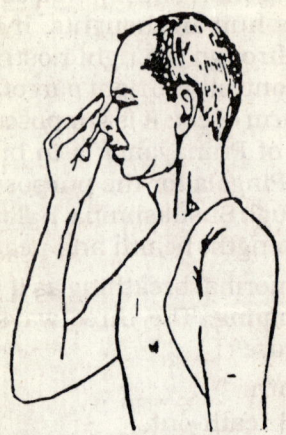

Fig. 7.8 : Pooraka through left nostril.

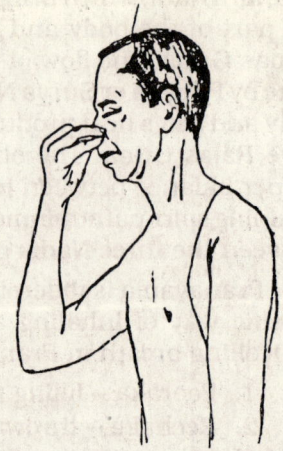

Fig. 7.9 : Baahya Kumbhaka.

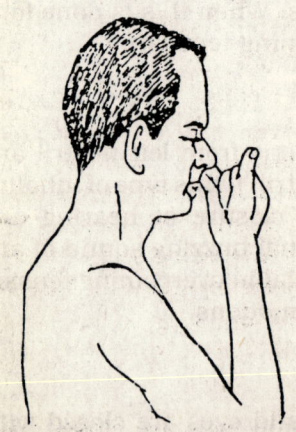

Fig. 7.10 : Pooraka (filling in the breath) through right nostril.

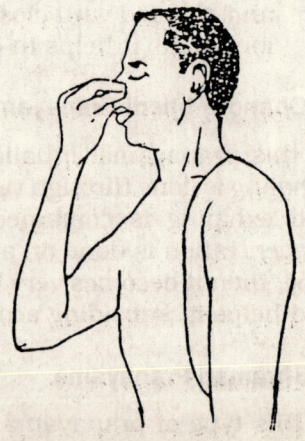

Fig. 7.11 : Aantarik Kumbhaka (Rolding in the breath)

antrik khumbaka and exhaling is done afterwards by slowly producing the buzzing sound of a Bhramar (i.e. bee). This pranayama strengthens the tissues of the brain and keeps the mind alert. This is very useful in relieving the tension.

4. Nadi Shodhan Pranayama

Purification of subtle perception paths. This pranayama, as the name suggests, helps in purifying the nerves and thereby strengthens the nervous system.

This pranayama is done in a comfortable sitting posture, breathing is done in a normal way. First, right nostril is closed and slow inhaling of air is done by left nostril. When the full breath is taken in left nostril is closed or breath is retained inside by doing antrik khumbaka for a few seconds. After lifting the thumb from the right nostril exhaling is done slowly by keeping the left nostril closed. After this, similar process is done by inhaling from right nostril retaining the breath inside exhaling from left nostril. This makes one round of Nadi Shodhana. It is important to remember the ratio of inhaling, retaining and exhaling of breath which for beginners is 1 : 2 : 2 and later on 1 : 4 : 2 : is considered to be ideal. The secret behind wonderful effects of this pranayama is that one holds one's breath in antrik khumbaka, the intake of fresh and pure air purifies lungs and when one throw the breath out (i.e. Bahya Khumbaka) then the cells of the lungs contract to squeeze out the impure air. In simple breathing, the pure air which one inhales is being exhaled immediately and as such pure air is not completely utilised in the body.

This pranayama produces the most favourable effect on nervous system and lungs.

5. Sheetli Pranayama (Beak Tongue Pranayama)

This pranayama is done in a comfortable pose. First of all, tongue is brought out, its edges are turned inside to give it the shape of a drain. This is done to avoid the entry of any foreign substance into the body as this is the only pranayama where inhaling of air is done through mouth by making a hissing sound. The antrik khumbaka is performed with all three bandhas. After this, bandhas, are released – first uddiyan, then jallandhar and then moolbandha and lastly exhaling is done through nose.

This pranayama produces a cooling effect on body and mind. If it is practised regularly, it is useful in changing the temperament of a person in a positive direction. The beneficial effect of this pranayama is also on blood purification level.

6. Kapal-bhati Pranayama

In this pranayama an effort is made to force out all the breath that one has inside and normal inhaling process is done. Initially an attempt is made to breath out 15-20 times without consciously taking breath inside. After this, breath is retained outside for few moments by doing bakya kumbaka. This is combined with mool bandha, the jallandhar bandha and uddiyan bandha. After bandhas are removed and normal inhaling of breath is done. This pranayama is particularly useful in purifying the impurities of nerves of the skull region and helps in controlling the sense organs. It is very useful in bringing relaxation of mind.

One has two types of energy i.e. Prana and Ayama. Prana energy controls various functions of the body above navel and is termed as positive force. Ayama energy controls the various functions of the body below navel. In moolbandha, prana shakti is moved upwards by lifting the rectum up. In uddhiyanbandha this prana shakti is pushed spine. In Jallandharbandha, ayama shakti is pushed down. Miraculous results can be achieved by the union of prana and ayama shaktis of the spine point behind navel.

Bandhas are safety-locks which are necessary to practice at the time of breath-retention for getting optimum utilization of oxygen that one inhales. For increasing tension-bearing capacity bandhas produce good results by calming down the agitated feelings. Mudras and bandha has serve to control and guide the psychic and pranic forces engendered or set in motion. To practice pranayama without bandhas can be disastrous. They perform the function that a transformer/fuse dose in circuit of electricity current. This bandhas play a protective role in avoiding pranic short-circuits in the body. The three bandhas which help in tension reduction. These are:

(a) Mula bandha (Anus-lock)

(b) Uddiyana Bandha (Fly-up lock)

(c) Jallandhar Bandha (Glottis-lock)

(a) Mula Bandha (Anus-Lock)

The essential elements of this bandha are
1. Simultaneous and continuous contraction of the internal and external anal sphincters.
2. Contraction of muscles lifting the anus.
3. Contraction of pelric floor.
4. Contraction of the lower abdomen to push back the viscera towards the sacrum.

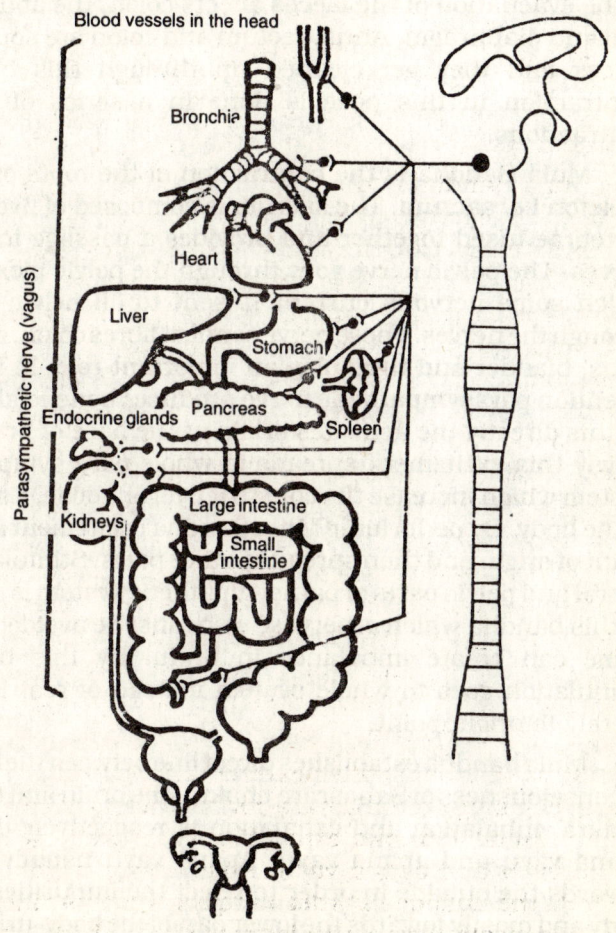

Fig. 7.12 : Mula Bandha

Efficiency of Mula Bandha depends on contraction of two sphincters that close the anus. There is external anal sphincter which closes the extremity of the digestive tract but it is essential that the second muscular ring, which is internal and lies two/three centimetres above in rectum must also be contracted. Contraction is done first in external and then on internal anal sphincter which leads to the contraction of the whole anal area and of the perineum. The contraction of the second sphincter plays an important role in the evacuation of the faeces affects colon, the abdominal wall and diaphragm. Anus, rectum and colon are sources of illness and they get cleaned up through this bandha. Contraction in this pose is done in a series of twenty contractions.

Mula Bandha is the contraction of the roots of whole skeleton i.e. sacrum. The sacrum is composed of five sacral vertebrae fused together and provides a passage to sacral nerves. The pelvic nerve goes through the pelvic plexu from which some nervous current is sent to all pelvic organs through the nerves. These nerve connect fibres colon, rectum, anus, bladder and thus play an important role. In breath-retention parasympathetic nerve produces beneficial effects as this directly the activates origin at the base of brain and slowly this excitement spreads to whole para sympathetic system which increase the constructive, anabolic, functions of the body. By performing Mula Bandha excitement is at the point of origin and then spread to other parts. Stimulation at sacral and pelvic parts of parasympathetic system is avoided in this bandha which otherwise also must be avoided as the same can create imbalance in brain. By this bandha, stimulation goes to whole system instead of restricting it merely to origin point.

Mula bandha establishes direct line between the centres of consciousness of Sahasrara chakra, the brain and the root chakra. Inhalation and exhalation is respectively done by prana vayu and apana vayu. Apana vayu usually moves towards the outside in order to reject the impurities of the body and mostly towards the lower part of the body-urination, defaecation, ejaculation, menstruation and child birth. During breath retention when Mula Bandha is combined with

Jallandhara Bandha the strong pranic current is generated. This energising current created at the base level rises along the susukshmna in the direction of sahasrara chakra.

This bandha helps in giving strength to inner muscles and activate their functioning. It has a very beneficial effect on the nervous system which increases the capacity of a person to bear tension producing factors.

(b) Uddiyana Bandha

During its practise one has the feeling that the stomach rises, literally 'flies away' upward. This bandha, like Mulla Bandha, must be practised on an empty stomach and the most propitious time is after the morning asana session. Lean slightly forward, place your hands on your thighs, above the knees or close to the groin, and empty your lungs completely (the weight of the torso must rest on the arms). Then raise the diaphragm by false inhalation; the intestines are forced back towards the spine as the abdomen retracts. Hold it for a few seconds, then release the bandha and inhale again. Mula Bandha and Uddiyana Bandha complete each other, since the organs concerned are closely related and perfectly synchronised. One should practise these bandhas together. After learning and mastering them separately they should be combined as a single exercise.

(c) Jalandhar Bandha

The best results are obtained by combining the three bandhas, that is by adding Jalandhara Bandha. When the lungs are filled with air, the ribs are lifted (which causes the thorax to expand), the neck is lowered until the chin exerts pressure on the body. To practise these bandhas, it is desirable to choose a quiet place where one will not be disturbed. When one practise the bandhas separately one must always concentrate on the muscles one is contracting whereas, if the three bandhas are combined, one must first concentrate on Mula Bandha, then on Uddiyana Bandha which is next, and finally on Jalandhara Bandha. Remain concentrated on the three bandhas. When they arre released (in reverse order : first Jalandhara, then Uddiyana, finally Mula Bandha) concentrate on each bandha as it relaxes.

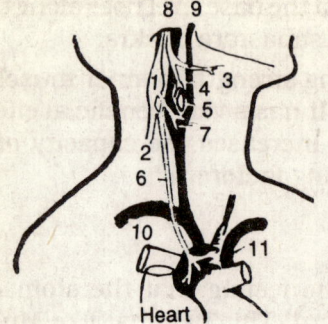

1. plexiform ganglion
2. vagus or pneumogastric nerve
3. glossopharyngeal nerve
4. carotid sinus nerve
5. intercarotid plexus
6. cardiocervical ramifications
7. carotid sinus
8. internal carotid artery
9. external carotid artery
10. subclavian artery
11. aorta

Fig. 7.13 : Jalandhara Bandha

MUDRAS

All diseases produce tension and mudras help in overcoming various problems leading to tension. Human body is consisted of five elements i.e. fire, air, earth, water and ether. The characteristics of fire.

These five elements are present in our body in the form of five sense organs other has the characteristic of sound, which we hear with out ears. The characteristic of air is touch, which we feel through skin. The characteristic of fire is light, which we feel with our eyes. The characteristic of water is taste, which we feel with our tongue. And similarly the characteristic of earth is smell, which we experience through our nose2

All diseases produces tension and Mudras technique helps in overcoming such problem produced by diseases. Our body is considered to be consisted of five elements :

(a) Fire
(b) Air
(c) Ether
(d) Earth
(e) Water.

All these elements mentioned above are represented in different fingers of our both hands. Thumbs of both hands represent 'fire' element, first finger represent 'air' element, second finger represent ether (sky) element, third finger from thump represent 'earth' element' and last finger represent 'water' element.

Mudras represent different poses of different fingers of the hands whereby different pressure is created on fingers which has the effect of increasing the speed of the cleaning processes of different elements present in these fingers.

1. GYAN MUDRA (First Finger and Thumb)

In this Mudra upper portion of thumb of hand is pressed with the upper portion of first finger. The pressure created, represent unification of 'fire' and 'air' element. When pressure is created on the upper portion of thumb, this has the effect of subsidising the agitated feelings. This pressure besides affecting 'Gyan Kendra' has the direct effect on pitutary and pineal gland. This mudra has direct effect on mental faculties. It smoothens the agitated feelings created by anger. It removes uncertainty, anger, fear and tension created therefrom. It strengthens nervous system.

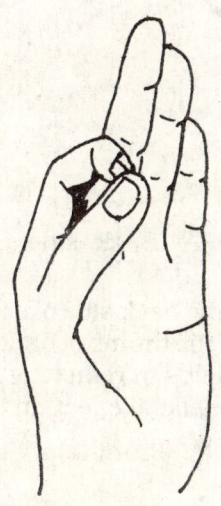

Fig. 7.14 : Gyan Mudra

2. VAYU MUDRA (Back side of first finger and thumb)

In this mudra, first finger is bend towards palm and pressure is given on the back side of this finger by thumb. This mudra has remarkable beneficial effect in removing the diseases of artharitis, paralysis, trembling etc. When this mudra is combined with 'aapan mudra' then it has the direct effect in removing the diseases relating to heart, thyroid gland.

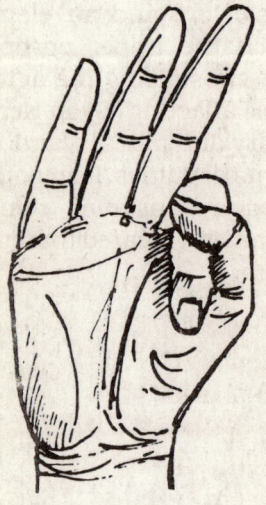 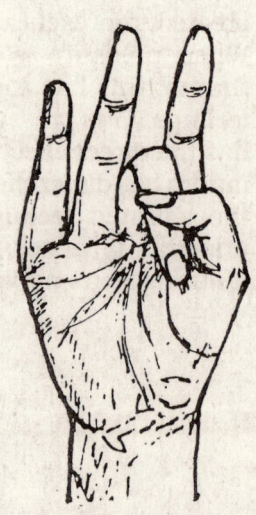

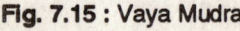

Fig. 7.15 : Vaya Mudra   **Fig. 7.16 :** Shunya Mudra

3. SHUNYA MUDRA (Back side of second finger and thumb)

In this mudra, the back side of second finger is pressed towards palm of the thumb of hand. Continuous practice of this mudra helps in removing hearing problem, and it has direct beneficial effect on thyroid gland.

4. PRITHVI MUDRA (Front top tip of third finger and thumb)

In this mudra, the upper portion of third finger front tip is pressed with the upper portion of thumb. This mudra helps in removing those diseases and increases capacity

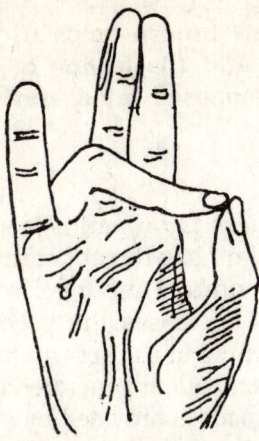

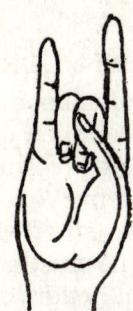

Fig. 7.17 : Prithvi Mudra   **Fig. 7.18 :** Aapaan Mudra

of body to increase capacity of the body to combat with diseases that spread due to deficiency of 'earth' element. It removes weakness of body, deficency of vitamins and helps in creating balance in body.

5. AAPAAN MUDRA (Middle two finger and thumb)

In this mudra second and third finger from thumb is pressed towards palm by the pressure created on the back side of these fingers by the thumb. This mudra helps in cleaning the body and in creating sattvic (positive) feelings. This mudra helps in removing blockage in urinary track.

6. PRANA MUDRA (Pressure by tips of last two fingers and thumb)

In this mudra, last two fingers of the hand is pressed on its tips by the upper portion of the thumb. This mudra has direct effect in increasing the visibility power.

7. SHAANT MUDRA

In this mudra, second finger from thumb presses the base of nose and the rest of three fingers only touches the nose. In this mudra, only light pressure is created by

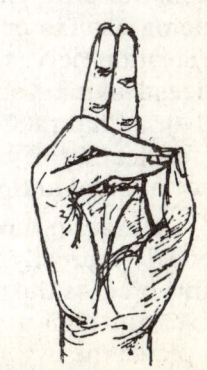

Fig. 7.19 : Prana Mudra

these fingers on the nose. This mudra helps in subsidising the agitated feelings and the feeling of anger is replaced by calm and composed mind and feelings.

8. LEKHNI MUDRA

Lekhni is boon from the Goddess Saraswati. When we hold pen then pressure on thumb has direct bearing in creating pressure on 'Budhi Kendra'. First finger which represent 'Vayu' (Air) element increases the speed of `Arash' (ether) element represented in the second finger and this process also give shelter to ideas generated from 'Budhi Kendra' i.e. ground element is provided by earth represented by third finger. This process also effect the water element represented by fourth finger from thumb which basically give flow to these ideas like flow of water.

Different Mudras effects different elements represented in different fingers of hand. Each mudra in itself helps in removing tension created in body different due to deficiency of these elements.

CONCENTRATION ON CHAKRAS – Tension Reduction Technique

The literal meaning of 'Chakra' is wheel. As per Tantra Yoga, there exist seven subtle Chakras in our body out of which five exist in spine, sixth in the forehead in the centre of the eyebrows and seventh at the back of the head at Brahmarandhra. Concentration of these Chakras at the time of doing asanas or at the time of meditation leads to the purification nerves and nerves fibres. Persons with unstable and restless mind should cooncentrate on Mooladhar Chakra and Ajna Chakra. Concentrating on different Chakras helps in purification of body and mind, which helps in getting peace of mind and remove tension.

Relaxation through concentration of Chakras is based affected by directly affected on our Central Nervous System. In this process the primordial energy 'Kundalini' situated in the sacrum bone at the base of spine on being activated rises up, pierce the five subtle Chakras and then unites with the all prevading cosmic energy after piercing Sahasrara Chakra

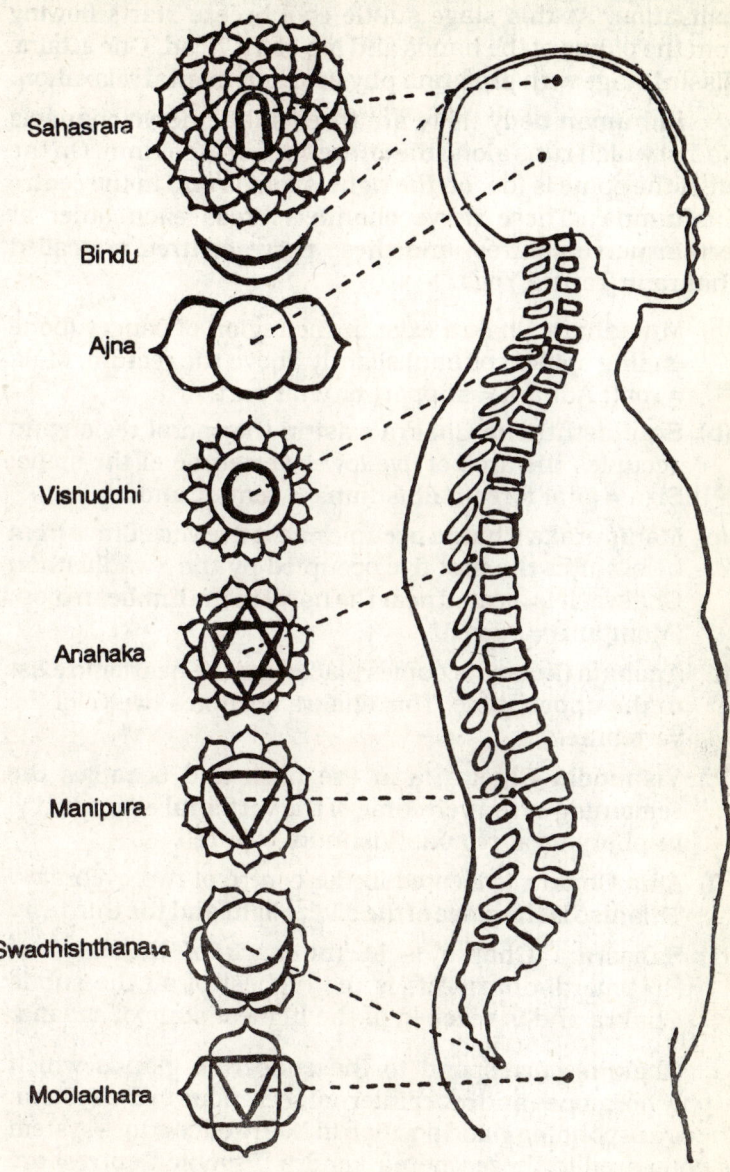

Fig. 7.22 : Position of chakras in human body.

at the top of the head. This stage is known as the stage of self realisation. At this stage subtle cool breeze starts flowing from the palms of the hands and top of the head. One attains blissful stage with profound physical and mental relaxation.

In human body there are three subtle nerve channels (Nadis) which runs along the entire vertebral column. On the left of the spine is Ida, on the right is Pingla and in the centre 'Sushumna'. These nerve channels cross each other at certain nerve centres, and these nerve centres are called Chakra in Tantra Yoga.

(a) Muladhara Chakra exist in the region of conccy (bone ending spinal column) slightly above the rectum. Mula = root; Adhara = support or vital part.

(b) Svadhisththana Chakra exist in the sacral region and occupies the area of five lower vertebrae of the spine. Sixa = vital force; Adhisthana = seat or ahode.

(c) Manipuraka Chakra occupies next five vertebrave from below after the first five occupied by the Swadhisthan Chakra. It is located near the navel in the lumber region. (Manipura = Navel).

(d) Anahata Chakra occupies place near the heart and exist in the upper spine. This chakra occupies twelve of the vertebrae.

(e) Vishuddhi Chakra is in the neck and occupies the remaining seven vertebrae of the vertebral column. It is in pharyngeal region. (Vishuddi = pure).

(f) Ajna Chakra is located in the centre of two eyebrows. This also is the place of the divine light and the third eye.

(g) Sahasrara Chakra is at the back of the head at Brahmarandhra. This is the highest of all the subtle Chakra and is reached in the highest state of sadana.

Chakras correspond to the endocrme glands which supply hormones and other internal secretious to the system. The corresponding gland position in Neuro endocrines system as compared to these Chetna-kendra (Psychic Centres) are as follows :

Psychic Centres		Neuro-Endocrine System
(a)	Jnankendra	Pineal Gland
(b)	Darshan Kendra	Pituitary Gland
(c)	Vishudhi Kendra	Thyroid Gland
(d)	Anand Kendra	Thymus Gland
(e)	Taijas Kendara	Pancreas
(f)	Swasthya Kendra	Andrenals Gland
(g)	Shakti Kendra	Gonads Gland

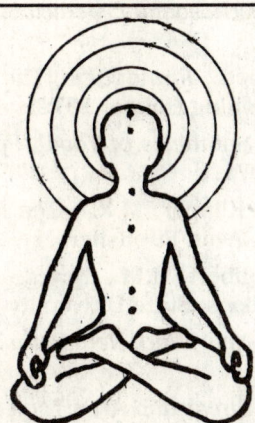

Neuro-Endocrine System

Pineal
Gland
Pituitary gland
Thyroid gland
Thymus gland
Pancreas
Adrenal glands
Gonads glands

Psychic Centres

Janam kendra
Darshan kendra
Vishudhi kendra
Anand kendra
Taijas kendra
Swasthya kendra
Shakti kendra

Fig. 7.23 : The neuro-endocrine system and the psychic centres placed in the human body.

By concentrating on a particular gland or its corresponding Psychic Centres the powers of that gland can be controlled to get the desired result and this helps in getting rid of diseases and tension produced by these diseases.

SELECT BIBLIOGRAPHY

Alexander, F.: *Psychosomatic Medicine*, New York, W.W. Norton & Co., 1950.

Andre Van Lysebeth, *Pranayama, The Yoga of Breathing*, Delhi, Vikas Publishing House, 1979.

Aurobindo: *The Synthesis of Yoga* , Pondicherry, Sri Aurobindo Ashram, 1971.

Benson, H. with Klipper, M.Z. : *The Relaxation Response*, New York, 1975, Avon Publishers.

Brooks, C.M., Gilbert, J.M., Keveg, H.A. and Curtes, D.R. : *Neurosecretions.* State University, New York, 1962.

Brown, Barbara: *New Mind, New Body* . New York, Harper & Row, 1975.

Brown, Barbara: *Stress and Art of Biofeedback* . New York, Harper & Row, 1977.

Cannon, W.B.: *Bodily changes in pain, hunger, fear and rage* , New York, Appleton, 1929.

Eliot, R.S. (ed.): *Stress and the Heart,* New York, Fatura Publishing Co.. 1974.

Fanibunda, E.B.: *Vision of the Divine.* Shri Satya Sai Books and Publications, P.O. Prashanti Nilayam, A.P., 1981.

Freud, Sigmund: *Introductory Lectures on Psychoanalysis,* Middlesex, Penguin Books Ltd., 1975.

Gaarder, K.R. and Montogomery, P.S.: *Clinical Biofeedback, A procedural manual,* Baltimore, Williams and Wilkins, 1977.

Gopi Krishna,: *The Awakening of Kundalini.* E. P. Dutton & Co., New York,1975.

Groen, J.J.: *Psychosomatic Research,* New York, Mac Millan Co., 1964.

James Hewitt. *The Complete Yoga* . New York, Schocken Books, 1978.

Karanjia, R. K., *Kundalini Yoga*, Arnold-Heinemann, New Delhi, 1977.

Kurtsin, I. T.: *Theoretical Principles of Psychosomatic Medicine.* New York, John Wiley & Sons, 1976.

Levi, L.: *Emotions, their parameters and measurement.* New York, Raven Press Publishers, 1975.

Levi, Lenart: *Society, Stress and Disease* Vol. I, London, Oxford University, Press, 1971.

Levi, L.: *Stress, Sources, Management and Prevention,* New York, Liveright Publishing Corporation, 1967.

Mahesh Yogi: *The Science of Being and Art of Living,* London, International S.R.M. Publications, 1966.

Monks of Ramakrishna Order: *Meditation,* Madras, Sri Ramakrishna Math, 1975.

Motoyama, H.: *A psychophysiological study of Yoga.* Tokyo Institute of Religious Psychology, 1976.

Pelletier, K.R.: *Mind as healer, Mind as Slayer. A Holistic approach to preventing stress disorder,* New York, Dill Publishers CO., 1977.

Peter Russell, *The T.M. Technique,* London, Routledge and Kegan Paul, 1979.

Pierllot, R.A.: *Recent Research in Psychosomatics,* Basel, S. Karger, 1970.

Rohit Mehta, *The science of Meditation.* Delhi, Motilal Banarasidass. 1978.

Schultz, J. and Luthe, W.: *Autogenic training, A Psychophysiologic approach in Psychotherapy,* New York, Grune and Stratton, 1959.

Selye, H.: *The stress of Life,* New York, Mc Graw Hill Book Co., 1950.

Steven Rose: *The Conscious Brain Middlesex, Penguin Books Ltd. 1976.*

Swami Muktananda: Meditate, Ganeshpuri, Gurudev Siddhs Peeth. 1981.

Tenbergen, N.: *Etiology and stress disease, Science,* 185: 26, 1974.

Weiner, H.: *Psychobiology and Human disease,* New York, Elsevier, 1977.

Wolff, H. G.: *Stress and Disease.* Shringfield, Charles C. Thomas, 1953.

ADDITIONAL
SUPPLEMENTARY READINGS

1. Ader, R. (ed.) (1981) *Psychoneuroimmunology* New York: Academic Press.
2. Cooper, C.L. and Payne, R. (eds) (1980) *Current Concerns in Occupational Stress* Chichester: J. Wiley.
3. Dohrenwend, B.S. and Dohrenwend, B.P. (1974) *Stressful Life Events: Their Nature and Effects* New York: Wiley.
4. Dohernwned, B.S. and Dohernwend, B.P. (eds) 1981 *Stressful Life Events and their Contexts.* New York: Prodist.
5. Glass, D.C. (1977) *Behaviour Patterns, Stress and Coronary Disease* Hillsdale, New Jersey: Lawrence Erlbaum.
6. Goldberger, L. and Breznitz, S (eds) (1982) *Handbook of Stress* New York: Free Press.
7. Henry, J.P. and Stephens, P.M. (1977) *Stress, Health and the Social Environment : A Sociologic Approach to Medicine* New York: Springer-Verlag.
8. Institute of Medicine (1981) *Research on Stress and Human Health* Washington DC National Academy Press.
9. Kutash, I.L. and Schlesinger L.B. (1980) *Handbook on Stress and Anxiety* San Francisco, California: Jossey-Boss.
10. Lazarus, R.S. (1976) *Patterns of Adjustment* New York: McGraw-Hill.
11. Liponiski, Z.J., Lipsitt, D.R. and Whybron, P.C.(eds) (1977) *Psychosomatic Medicine: Current Trends and Clinical Applications* New York: Oxford University Press.
12. Mechanic, D.(ed) (1982) *Handbook of Health , Helath Care and the Health Profession* New York:Free Press.
13. Mc. Gaugh, J.L. and Kiesler, S.B. (eds) (1981) *Aging: Biology and Behaviour* New York: Academic Press.
14. Ojeman, R.G. (ed) (1959) *Recent Contributions of Biological and Psychosocial Investigations to Preventive Psycliatry* Iowa City, State University Iowa.
15. Selye, H (1974) *Stress Without Distress* Philadelphia; Pennsylvania : Lippin Cott.
16. Selye, H. (1950) *The Physiology and Pathology of Exposure to Stress.* Montreal: Acta
17. Selye, H. (1980) (ed) *Selye's Guide to Stress Research.* New York: Van Nostrand Reinhold.
18. Weiss, S.M., Hard, J.A. and Fox, B.H. (eds) (1981) *Prespectives on Behavioural Medicine* New York: Academic Press.